GW01091202

Understanding
INFERTILITY

Peter G. Wardle &
David J. Cahill

Published by Family Doctor Publications Limited
in association with the British Medical Association

IMPORTANT NOTICE

This book is intended not as a substitute for personal medical advice but as a supplement to that advice for the patient who wishes to understand more about his/her condition.

Before taking any form of treatment YOU SHOULD ALWAYS CONSULT YOUR MEDICAL PRACTITIONER.

In particular (without limit) you should note that advances in medical science occur rapidly and some of the information about drugs and treatment contained in this booklet may very soon be out of date.

Family Doctor Publications, 10 Butchers Row, Banbury, Oxon OX16 8JH

Medical Editor: Dr Tony Smith
Consultant Editor: Victoria Gilbert
Cover Artist: Dave Eastbury
Medical Artist: Peter Cox Associates
Design: MPG Design, Blandford Forum, Dorset
Printing: Reflex Litho, Thetford, using acid-free paper

ISBN: 1 898205 53 1

Contents

Introduction

Most adults intend to have children. If you have picked up this book, it is likely that you, a member of your family or a close friend is having difficulties in achieving this aim. You are not alone. Fertility problems are probably the most common reason (other than pregnancy) for anyone between the ages of 20 and 45 seeking medical advice in this country. About a quarter of all couples will experience an unexpected delay in achieving the size of family they want, and most of these will consult their GP. About a sixth of all couples will be seen at a hospital fertility clinic.

The aim of this book is to help you to understand more about getting pregnant, why you may not have been successful so far, the investigations and tests that may be needed to establish the cause, and the infertility treatments available.

Infertility is more than just a medical or physical problem. It can also lead to intense emotional and psychological distress. This can disrupt a couple's relationship with each other and with friends, family and work colleagues who may seem to be achieving parenthood very easily. The world around such couples seems a fertile place from which they are excluded, and they may even withdraw from social situations where they may meet pregnant women or young children. Most clinics recognise the emotional aspects of infertility, and include specially trained counsellors among their staff. However, some couples are reluctant to seek this type of professional support. This book therefore includes a chapter on coping with infertility.

Infertility and its various treatments raise moral concerns and ethical dilemmas for many couples. This is particularly the case for new assisted conception treatments, egg and sperm donation, and surrogacy. These are important issues but beyond the scope of a small book like this, and we deal with them only briefly.

Doctors, nurses and scientists often use technical medical terms. You may be unfamiliar with a number of these words, so there is an explanatory glossary at the end of the book. The glossary also includes explanations of acronyms (such as IUI, GIFT and ICSI) and abbreviations that are commonly used in infertility tests and treatments.

A small book of this type has to be concise. We have included a list of information sources for couples who would like more detail on pages 82–4.

KEY POINTS

✓ Fertility problems are a very frequent reason for people to seek medical advice

✓ About a quarter of all couples will experience an unexpected delay in achieving the size of family that they want

✓ Approximately a sixth of all couples will visit a hospital fertility clinic for advice

✓ Infertility is more than just a medical or physical problem; it can also lead to intense emotional and psychological distress

What is infertility?

Absolute infertility, or sterility, with no chance of natural conception is very rare. It occurs only if, for example, the man is not producing sperm, the woman has had a premature menopause and has no eggs remaining in her ovaries, or both of the woman's fallopian tubes are blocked (preventing sperm from reaching her eggs). These problems can often be overcome with fertility treatments.

Most fertility problems, however, are in fact low fertility, or subfertility, where a couple has been trying to conceive for some time without success. How long is 'some time'? This depends on a number of factors, particularly the woman's age and whether there are other reasons to suspect a fertility problem.

Most of us were told as teenagers, by well-meaning parents and teachers, that getting pregnant was very easy unless we used a reliable form of contraception. In fact, compared with most other animal species, humans have relatively poor natural fertility. In young fertile couples, the highest chance of conceiving in each monthly cycle, when they first start to try, is only 33 per cent (one in three), or throwing a six with two dice.

For most couples, the chance of conceiving is lower than this, on average a one in five or six chance

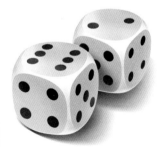

For young fertile couples, the chance of conceiving may be as high as one in three (33 per cent), or throwing a six with two dice.

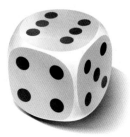

For most couples, the chance of conceiving is on average one in six (17%), or throwing a six with one dice.

each month – about the same chance as throwing a six with a dice.

Just like throwing a six, the chance of pregnancy increases with the number of monthly cycles a couple has been trying. Fifty per cent of couples who are fertile will have conceived by three months, 75 per cent by six months and 90 per cent by twelve months. By two years, this has increased only slightly to 95 per cent.

In general, you should consult your doctor if you have not conceived within one year of trying, and certainly after two years. However, this does not take account of the woman's age. A woman's natural fertility starts to reduce from her late 20s – slowly at first, more rapidly after the age of 35 and very sharply after the age of 40. This is mainly a result of the reduction in the quality of the eggs remaining in her ovaries.

Not only does a woman's chance of achieving a pregnancy decrease as she gets older, but also her risk of miscarriage increases if she does conceive. This is probably related to the quality of her eggs and the resulting embryo rather than any problem with the lining of her uterus. In addition, the risk of conceiving a child affected by a chromosome abnormality (such as Down's syndrome) rises progressively after a woman reaches the age of 35. Therefore, if the woman is over 35, couples should seek expert advice promptly if they have not conceived within one year. If the woman has reached 40 years of age, they should seek advice after six months.

There are many other reasons why some couples should seek help even earlier. For the man, this may be a past infection of his testes (orchitis) or surgery (perhaps to correct the failure of his testes to descend properly into his scrotum in childhood). For the woman, this may be irregular or infrequent periods, previous pelvic infection, severe appendicitis or abdominal surgery (perhaps to remove an ovarian cyst). For more on this, see 'Why can't we conceive?' on page 17.

SEEKING ADVICE

Some couples delay seeking medical advice because they are finding it difficult to accept that they may have a problem or because they are concerned that they will be asked questions about personal and private aspects of their lives. Your GP and the staff at a fertility clinic will be aware of these feelings. They are familiar with the anxieties and fears about the investigations, the problems that they may find and the treatment options. The information that they will give you will enable you to decide whether and how you wish to proceed. Delay in seeking advice may limit the treatment options that may be available or their chance of success.

Even if you seek medical advice because of infertility, it does not necessarily follow that you will need any treatment to improve your chance of pregnancy. Some couples find that they have conceived while waiting for a clinic appointment or during the course of their blood tests and other investigations. Many others find that the results of the various tests are all normal. If you have been trying to conceive for a relatively short time, you may simply be reassured by the clinic that your chance of pregnancy remains high, and you may be advised to return for a review appointment if you have not been successful after a few more months. In addition, some investigations, such as those to check that your fallopian tubes are open, may temporarily enhance fertility.

You may be concerned that all you will be offered are expensive, high-technology infertility treatments, such as in vitro fertilisation (IVF). This is understandable given the huge amount of media interest that these treatments have attracted. However, many of the potential causes of infertility can be corrected with much simpler treatments, such as drug therapy.

IS INFERTILITY ON THE RISE?

The brief answer is no. However, there has been a large increase in the number of couples seeking specialist help over the past 15 years. This is partly because there is now a greater awareness about the increasing range and effectiveness of infertility treatments. The increased media attention has made infertility less of a taboo, which means that friends and acquaintances may be more open in talking about their own experiences of fertility problems.

Many couples now delay having children. This may be for the woman to pursue her career, or for a couple to achieve greater financial stability or pursue other ambitions before having a family. Twenty-five years ago, the average age for a woman to have her first child was in her early 20s, a decade ago it was 25 years, now it is 28 years. This delay, to an age at which the woman's natural fertility is starting to reduce, inevitably means that more couples will experience difficulty in conceiving and will seek medical advice. Research from the USA shows that, in more than half the couples seen at infertility clinics, the woman is over 35. By this age, natural fertility is reducing rapidly, and many couples may need to consider more effective (but also more stressful and expensive) high-technology treatments to optimise their chance of pregnancy.

The question of whether men's fertility is declining is also important. There have been several reports recently in the media and scientific press suggesting that sperm counts are falling. Some of these have looked at results over time and have found a fall in overall sperm numbers. Others have found no change, and some have even found an increase within their own laboratory. It may be that, as examination techniques have become more rigid, the actual sperm counts being reported are lower.

On the other hand, the reported trends may reflect a real fall in sperm numbers, possibly as a result of toxins (poisons) in the environment and the increasing use of steroid hormones in food production. At present, the scientific community does not believe there is any great cause for concern, as the evidence for a reduction in sperm counts is not particularly strong. However, this issue is not yet resolved.

KEY POINTS

✓ Infertility is a common problem, affecting at least one in six couples at some time in their lives

✓ Most couples with infertility have low fertility rather than sterility

✓ Ninety per cent of normal fertile couples will conceive within a year

✓ Couples who have not conceived within one or two years should seek medical advice

✓ The woman's age is the most important predictor of a couple's fertility

✓ Women over 35 years should seek advice if they have not conceived within one year at the most

✓ Couples should seek medical advice earlier if the woman has infrequent periods or the man has had previous surgery or an infection involving his testes

Getting pregnant

To understand the problem of infertility, you need to know what is normal. It may seem obvious to some people how their body works, particularly the parts to do with sexual activity and childbirth. But getting pregnant is more than just having sexual intercourse or the joining of a sperm with an egg. The process is actually quite complex.

FEMALE FERTILITY

Every month, an egg is released from one of a woman's two ovaries, as part of her menstrual cycle. This is controlled by hormones formed in the brain, the pituitary gland (at the base of the brain), and the ovaries themselves. In most women, the menstrual cycle is regular and lasts about 28 days.

The main female hormones are: gonadotrophin-releasing hormone (GnRH), which is produced in the hypothalamus at the centre of the brain; follicle-stimulating hormone (FSH) and luteinising hormone (LH), which are produced in the pituitary; and oestrogen and progesterone, which are produced in the ovaries.

At the beginning of the menstrual cycle, the levels of oestrogen and progesterone are low and GnRH stimulates the secretion of FSH from the pituitary. FSH in turn stimulates an egg to grow within a follicle (a fluid sac) inside one of the ovaries. In each menstrual cycle, around ten small egg follicles reach the size and stage of maturity at which they could respond to FSH. However, usually only one will become the major or dominant follicle in that cycle, the one destined to ovulate. All the others will die off.

As the dominant follicle grows, it produces increasing amounts of oestrogen, which enters the bloodstream. Oestrogen has a direct action on the lining of the

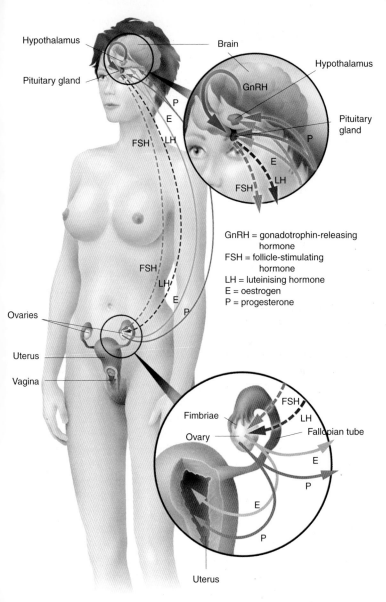

GnRH = gonadotrophin-releasing hormone
FSH = follicle-stimulating hormone
LH = luteinising hormone
E = oestrogen
P = progesterone

Every month, an egg is released from one of a woman's two ovaries, as part of her menstrual cycle. This is controlled by hormones formed in the brain, the pituitary gland and the ovaries themselves.

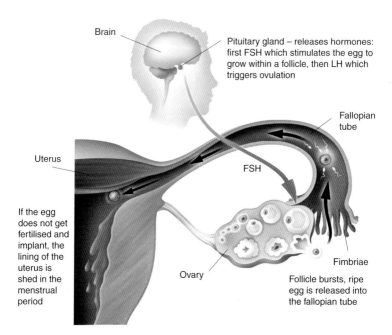

Brain

Pituitary gland – releases hormones:
first FSH which stimulates the egg to
grow within a follicle, then LH which
triggers ovulation

Fallopian
tube

Uterus

FSH

If the egg
does not get
fertilised and
implant, the
lining of the
uterus is
shed in the
menstrual
period

Ovary

Fimbriae

Follicle bursts, ripe
egg is released into
the fallopian tube

The menstrual cycle is typically 28 days; for the first 14 days the egg matures in the ovary
before being released into the fallopian tube at ovulation. If the ripe egg is unfertilised,
the lining of the uterus is shed in the menstrual period about 14 days after ovulation.

uterus or womb (the endometrium),
making it thicker in preparation for a
possible pregnancy. After about
10–12 days, when oestrogen levels
in the bloodstream reach a critical
level, the pituitary releases a
sudden surge of another hormone,
LH, which acts on the follicle and
the egg to prepare them for
ovulation. LH reaches its peak in the
bloodstream within a few hours and
triggers ovulation within about 36
to 42 hours. At ovulation, the
follicle bursts, releasing the ripe egg
into the fallopian tube.

After ovulation, the follicle walls
collapse and mature into a small
mass of yellow tissue, which begins
to produce progesterone as well as
oestrogen. Progesterone increases
the supply of blood to the
endometrium. The endometrium
becomes more succulent and
produces a sugar-rich compound,
glycogen, which can be used by a
developing embryo.

The egg can be fertilised for 24
hours after ovulation. If it meets
sperm in the fallopian tube, then
fertilisation is likely to occur. If the

egg remains unfertilised, or if it fertilises but fails to implant in the uterus, the endometrium is shed as the menstrual period about 14 days after ovulation.

MALE FERTILITY

A man's testes have two main functions: to make the major male sex hormone, testosterone, and to produce sperm. The production of sperm is mainly controlled by the hormone FSH and testosterone production is mainly regulated by LH, the same hormones that control egg production in a woman. In men, LH is sometimes called by another name, interstitial cell-stimulating hormone (ICSH). FSH acts on tissues in the testes called the seminiferous tubules, which are the main areas of sperm cell production. LH acts on other cell types in the testes that produce testosterone, the main hormone responsible for hair growth, muscular build and virility.

Sperm production is a more lengthy process than the production of an egg. However, in contrast to egg production, where the eggs have been present since birth, sperm production occurs from cells of very recent origin, not more than six months old. The sperm cells produced in the seminiferous tubules are not capable of fertilisation. They mature as they pass through the epididymis (a narrow system of tiny tubes on the surface of the testes). Mature sperm, which are capable of fertilisation, can be found in the vas deferens (a thin cord-like structure above the testes). It takes between three and four months for sperm to develop from the immature stages within the seminiferous tubules to mature sperm within the vas deferens. During this time, sperm production may be affected by several factors, including any illness that causes a fever or exposure to substances that are toxic to sperm, such as some industrial chemicals or use of recreational drugs, such as those used for body building.

At ejaculation, powerful contractions occur in the urethra (the tube within the penis that carries urine and semen to the outside of the body), the seminal vesicles (which secrete seminal fluid) and the ejaculatory ducts. These force the sperm and seminal fluid out of the urethra in spurts. If the penis is in the vagina at the time, the force carries the sperm up to the woman's cervix (the neck of her uterus). About 100 million sperm are ejaculated, and one million may swim into the cervical mucus. The sperm then swim through the mucus secretions in the cervix and uterus and out along the fallopian tubes, a journey that takes about 12 hours. Only about 500 to 1,000 sperm remain by the time

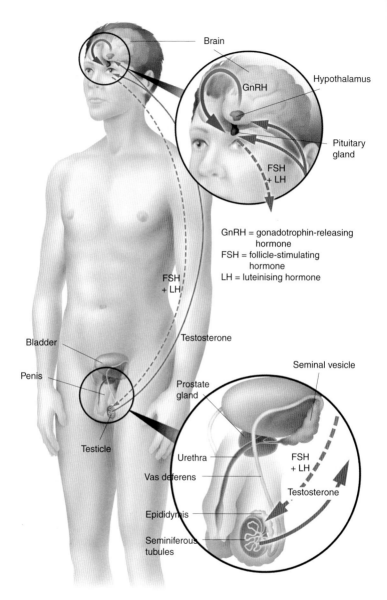

Brain

GnRH

Hypothalamus

Pituitary gland

FSH + LH

GnRH = gonadotrophin-releasing hormone
FSH = follicle-stimulating hormone
LH = luteinising hormone

FSH + LH

Testosterone

Bladder

Penis

Prostate gland

Seminal vesicle

Urethra

Vas deferens

FSH + LH

Testosterone

Epididymis

Testicle

Seminiferous tubules

A man's testes have two main fuctions: to make testosterone and to produce sperm. Sperm production is mainly controlled by the hormone FSH, and testosterone production is mainly regulated by LH. Both FSH and LH are produced in the pituitary gland.

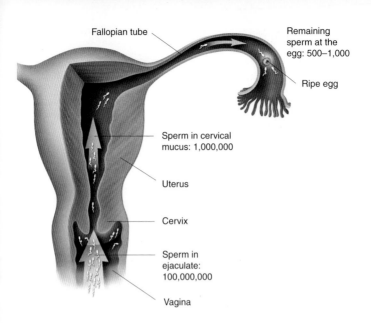

Of about 100 million sperm that are ejaculated, only around 500 to 1,000 remain by the time they reach the egg at the outer end of the fallopian tube.

they reach the egg at the outer end of the fallopian tube which is where fertilisation normally occurs.

The sperm make this journey largely under the power of their own swimming ability. If the woman has an orgasm, contractions within her uterus provide some help. Sperm are able to survive for several days, much longer than an egg. They lie in wait at the outer end of the woman's fallopian tube at the time she ovulates. Although many sperm stick to the outside of an egg, only one is usually successful in actually penetrating the coverings of the egg to fertilise it. Multiple embryos result from either multiple eggs (oocytes) being fertilised in non-identical twins or triplets or from a fertilised egg splitting into two – identical twins.

AFTER CONCEPTION

If the egg is fertilised, it begins to divide rapidly (forming a morula) and is moved towards the uterus by the cilia (hairs) which are present in the lining of the fallopian tube. The cells of the fertilised egg initially divide without increasing the overall size of the embryo. The cells get smaller as they increase in number and remain in their surrounding 'egg shell', called the zona pellucida.

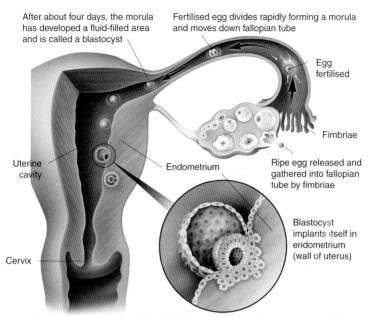

After about four days, the morula has developed a fluid-filled area and is called a blastocyst

Fertilised egg divides rapidly forming a morula and moves down fallopian tube

Egg fertilised

Fimbriae

Uterine cavity

Endometrium

Ripe egg released and gathered into fallopian tube by fimbriae

Cervix

Blastocyst implants itself in endometrium (wall of uterus)

The fertilised egg divides rapidly, first to form a morula and then a blastocyst. After about six to seven days, the blastocyst reaches the uterine cavity where it implants in the endometrium.

By the fourth day, the morula has developed a fluid-filled area in its centre and is now called a blastocyst which contains 32 to 64 cells. A small number of cells in the centre are destined to be the embryo; the remainder will make up the placenta (afterbirth) and other parts of the tissues that support the pregnancy.

At about day 6 or 7 after fertilisation, the developing blastocyst reaches the cavity of the uterus, hatches out of the zona pellucida and implants (embeds itself) into the endometrium. The placenta invades the mother's tissues and

develops a firm attachment and blood supply for the ongoing pregnancy.

THE EFFECT OF AGE

Male and female fertility are both affected by age. A woman's ovaries contain all her eggs from birth and no more eggs will be produced during her lifetime. With increasing age, and particularly once a woman reaches her 40s, the number of follicles and eggs available in her ovaries have decreased to a degree where conception becomes less likely.

When a woman reaches the

menopause, her ability to conceive is lost. At this time, her ovaries no longer contain any follicles capable of developing and maturing. However, her uterus is still capable of carrying a pregnancy, even after her own egg reserves have been exhausted. This has been demonstrated by well-publicised cases where women in their 50s and 60s have borne children as a result of treatment with donor eggs.

There are many tales of men fathering children into their 70s, and these are probably true. However, most men experience a gradual reduction in testosterone production and sperm production as they get older. They are also less able to sustain their erection to allow sexual intercourse. By 55 years, the quality of their sperm is considerably affected. There is also a steadily increasing risk of passing on chromosomal abnormalities such as Down's syndrome after this age.

INCREASING THE CHANCE OF CONCEPTION

The likelihood of conceiving depends on several factors. The younger the couple (particularly the woman), the higher the chance of success. The frequency of sexual intercourse is another important factor – if the frequency is consistently less than once weekly, a pregnancy is much less likely to occur. In addition, sexual intercourse needs to involve full vaginal penetration, so that sperm are deposited at the top of the vagina close to the cervix. However, for some couples, the time interval from trying to get pregnant to achieving a pregnancy may vary considerably without any obvious explanation.

✓ Each monthly cycle, a woman generally produces one egg capable of being fertilised

✓ The egg that is produced has been present in the woman's body since before birth

✓ At ejaculation, a man produces millions of sperm, although less than 1,000 ever reach the egg

✓ The sperm that are released have taken about three or four months to develop

✓ Fertility declines with age, after 35 years for women and after 55 years for men

✓ The likelihood of conception is increased by regular intercourse throughout the woman's monthly cycle, particularly during the seven to ten days after her period has finished

Why can't we conceive?

ELEMENT OF CHANCE

Most couples have unrealistically high expectations of how quickly they will conceive when they start trying for a family. For normal fertile couples, the monthly chance of conception varies between one in three (at the most) and about one in twenty, the average being about one in six. Many couples find it difficult to accept that chance has anything to do with achieving a pregnancy and that their failure to conceive may simply be the result of bad luck.

If we take the example of an average fertile couple with about a one in six monthly chance of pregnancy, we can compare this to the frustration of repeatedly failing to throw a six with a dice. The dice is not weighted against us, we are simply being unlucky. Of course, the more times a dice is thrown for a six unsuccessfully, the more likely it becomes that there is a problem

with the dice – that it is weighted against us. Or, in the case of pregnancy, that there is a fundamental problem reducing the chance of conception.

A couple throwing a 20-sided dice for a '20' is roughly equivalent to the lower limit of normal human fertility. After 24 throws, or two years of trying, there is about a 65 per cent chance of success, which increases to about 75 per cent after 36 throws or three years of trying. Very few couples have a zero chance of pregnancy and, even with a very small chance each month, it is possible that they will conceive in time. For example, even with a one in 100 chance each month, almost 30 per cent of couples would have achieved a pregnancy by three years.

For most infertile couples, their chance of conceiving naturally is likely to be unrealistically low by the time they are seen in a specialist

THE LIKELIHOOD OF CONCEIVING INCREASES WITH TIME

Monthly chance of pregnancy	Pregnant by 2 years	Pregnant by 3 years
1 in 5	94 per cent	97 per cent
1 in 20	64 per cent	76 per cent
1 in 100	21 per cent	29 per cent
1 in 500	5 per cent	7 per cent

clinic. Depending on whether a fertility problem is found and of what type, there are likely to be a number of options for treatment. Each treatment is likely to offer a different chance of success, but it is unreasonable to expect any of them to exceed the highest monthly chance for couples with normal fertility: about 33 per cent (one in three).

IS OVULATION OCCURRING?

If you have a regular monthly period (never more than one or two days early or late), you will almost always be releasing an egg from one of your ovaries. This usually occurs about 14 days before your period would be due to start. Many women are able to recognise the time of ovulation – they may experience low abdominal discomfort for a few hours on the side where an egg has just been released or may notice an increased amount of mucus discharge from

their vagina for a day or two beforehand. Women who have irregular or infrequent periods are likely to have a reduced chance of conceiving, and many may not be ovulating at all.

If your periods have been very regular in the past and have only become irregular fairly recently, this may be caused by being underweight, losing weight rapidly through dieting, emotional stress or too much exercise. Changing your lifestyle may be all that is necessary to correct this.

If your periods have always been irregular, or have become irregular with a steady increase in weight, you may have a condition called polycystic ovarian syndrome (PCOS). This is an inherited condition that can cause subfertility, irregular periods and possibly increase the risk of miscarriage. In PCOS, the ovaries contain many small benign (non-cancerous) cysts. The cysts are actually immature egg follicles and not true 'cysts'. They do not usually need to be removed by surgery, although this may be necessary if a large cyst develops.

PCOS causes a hormone imbalance, which can result in irregular ovulation, failure of ovulation, or a reduction in the quality of eggs that the woman releases from her ovaries. Other symptoms include an increased tendency to develop acne, an increased amount of body hair, an increased tendency to put on weight and difficulty in losing weight. Many women with PCOS need medical treatment. However, some find that, by losing weight, their menstrual cycle becomes more regular. This improves their chance of conception and reduces their risk of miscarriage. It may often help their other symptoms.

TIMING AND FREQUENCY OF INTERCOURSE

For the best chance of pregnancy, a couple should have sexual inter-course when the woman's cervical mucus is most receptive to sperm, usually one or two days before ovulation. Most women are aware that they produce more cervical mucus in the middle of their cycle. Their cervical mucus becomes clearer in appearance and more stretchy and fluid, rather like the raw white of a hen's egg. Some women will notice that they feel more damp at this time. A woman's sex drive may also be noticeably increased, as a result of hormonal changes around the time of ovulation. Some couples may use commercially available ovulation detection kits, which identify these hormone changes, to determine when the woman is ovulating.

It is not necessary for couples to focus their love-making solely around the time of ovulation. This can lead to difficulties in a couple's relationship, as both partners may start to feel that they are having to perform to a schedule. The timing

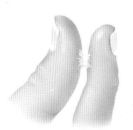
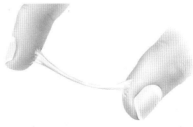

Non-receptive   Receptive

For the best chance of pregnancy, a couple should have sex when the woman's cervical mucus is most receptive to sperm. The mucus becomes clearer, stretchy and fluid – rather like the raw egg white of a hen's egg.

of intercourse is not particularly critical if a couple are having intercourse every two to four days. Once in the cervical mucus, sperm can survive for several days, possibly up to a week, and will retain their normal ability to fertilise an egg for most of this time. They gradually pass through the cervical mucus into the woman's uterus and along her fallopian tubes where, if they meet the egg, fertilisation normally occurs.

There is no evidence that a couple's chance of pregnancy is reduced by having intercourse too often. Although the volume of semen a man releases may be less, this is simply the result of a reduction in the fluid content. The number of functionally competent sperm remains virtually unchanged. There is also no evidence that the position of sexual intercourse makes pregnancy more or less likely. Neither does lying still for any period of time after sex or propping a pillow under the buttocks.

LIFESTYLE FACTORS

A number of lifestyle factors and past or current medical problems may reduce your chance of pregnancy. The main lifestyle factors to consider are smoking and alcohol.

Substances in cigarette smoke are toxic to eggs and sperm, and to the developing embryo in preg-nancy. Smoking by either partner reduces the chance of getting pregnant naturally or by fertility treatments, and there is increasing evidence that passive exposure to cigarette smoke may be almost as harmful. Smokers take about 30 per cent longer to achieve a pregnancy than non-smokers and, with IVF treatment, the proportion of eggs that fertilise will be 20 to 30 per cent lower. You should try to give up smoking while you are at an early stage of infertility investigations.

Heavy alcohol consumption can affect important hormone levels in men and women, and interfere with sperm production and sperm function. However, smaller amounts of alcohol do not seem to be damaging. It is sensible for you both to restrict your alcohol consumption to less than six units each week while you are trying for a pregnancy (one unit is equivalent to a half-pint of beer or a small glass of wine).

MEDICAL PROBLEMS

If you have experienced medical problems in the past, this can reduce your chance of getting pregnant, so seek advice early on. For the man, this may be because of a testicular infection (orchitis) or surgery in the past. Orchitis is most likely to damage sperm production if it is caused by a viral infection such as mumps. If it is caused by a bacterial infection, it may lead to scarring and obstruction of the vas deferens and epididymis. Previous surgery in the area around the testes can also damage these narrow tubes or restrict the blood circulation to the testes. Operations for childhood hernias, to correct any failure of the testes to descend properly into the scrotum or to treat the painful emergency of testicular torsion, are important indications to seek fertility advice early.

For the woman, any past gynaecological problems or pelvic infection may affect her fertility, as well as any previous pelvic or abdominal operations. Surgery causes scar tissue to form as part of the normal healing process and sometimes other tissues close by can be involved. For example, the fallopian tubes may become obstructed by scar tissue after severe appendicitis or surgery to remove an ovarian cyst.

Current medical problems may also reduce your fertility. Some of these (such as thyroid disease) are checked for during routine fertility investigations. For other medical conditions, such as diabetes or epilepsy, you may need to have an assessment before you try for a pregnancy. If in doubt, see your GP.

THE EFFECT OF MEDICATION

Various drugs can reduce your fertility. If you are taking medicines regularly, check with your GP, pharmacist or local fertility clinic before trying for a pregnancy. As a general rule, it is best to avoid all drugs that are not absolutely necessary while trying to conceive.

Drugs that can affect a man's fertility include sulphasalazine, which is used in the treatment of inflammatory bowel diseases, and some blood pressure treatments, such as beta-blockers and captopril (which can also cause impotence). Anti-malarial drugs may reduce sperm counts, as can the excessive use of simple pain-killers such as aspirin. Drug abuse can also reduce male fertility, particularly anabolic ('body-building') steroids and marijuana.

Drugs that reduce a woman's fertility usually do so by interfering with ovulation. Some affect a woman's normal hormone levels by increasing the production of the hormone prolactin. Although prolactin is an important hormone for the production of breast milk after pregnancy, it stops a woman having periods if she produces it excessively at other times. Drugs that can cause excessive prolactin production include various tranquillisers, sedatives and other treatments for minor psychiatric problems, as well as some anti-sickness drugs such as metoclopramide. A wide range of anti-inflammatory drugs and anti-arthritis drugs can reduce a woman's fertility by blocking ovulation. Examples of these are indomethacin, naproxen, diclofenac and mefenamic acid. Even aspirin or paracetamol can cause problems if they are taken in high doses. As in men, drug abuse will also reduce a woman's fertility, particularly marijuana, which can suppress the hormones follicle-stimulating hormone (FSH) and luteinising hormone (LH).

KEY POINTS

✓ Chance is an important factor in a couple's fertility

✓ Women with infrequent, irregular or absent periods should seek fertility advice early

✓ Being underweight or overweight can reduce a woman's fertility

✓ If a couple are having intercourse every two to four days, they should not need to worry about the best time to conceive

✓ Having intercourse very frequently does not reduce the chance of getting pregnant

✓ Couples trying to conceive should avoid smoking and passive smoking and restrict their alcohol consumption

✓ Seek medical advice about any drugs that you are taking to check that they are not reducing your fertility

Investigating infertility

WHEN SHOULD WE SEEK HELP?

The answer to this is not as simple as six months, 12 months or any particular length of time. The standard definition of infertility is the inability to conceive within one year of regular intercourse without the use of contraceptives. Most couples should seek medical help after one year. For many, it may even be appropriate to wait longer than that. Up to 90 per cent of normal fertile couples will be pregnant at the end of one year and up to 95 per cent by two years. However, couples with a complex problem or increasing age may need to seek help more rapidly than this. Initially a couple should see their own GP who will be able to assess their situation, arrange some of their preliminary tests and advise about whether referral to a local or specialist fertility clinic is indicated.

SHOULD WE USE THE NHS OR GO TO A PRIVATE CLINIC?

Most NHS clinics can provide a comprehensive range of basic investigations to establish why you can't conceive. They will also provide some fertility treatments such as tubal surgery or ovulation induction. Some do provide in vitro fertilisation (IVF), although the numbers treated may be limited by the funding available.

Private clinics generally provide a range of treatments – some are purely IVF centres whereas others provide full diagnostic and therapeutic services. The Human Fertility and Embryology Authority (HFEA) who are responsible for licensing all IVF clinics also provide information about successful pregnancy rates. When you are selecting a private fertility clinic, you need to find out the cost, the range of facilities that are available, whether you could be seen quickly or at unsocial hours, and the experience and qualifications of the doctor who will be seeing you.

There are several other ways of finding out information about private clinics. The decision to attend a particular clinic often depends on sheer practicalities, such as ease of access and location. If there are several clinics within driving distance, contact them first for the information leaflets or booklets that they will provide for prospective patients. Your GP or hospital consultant may also recommend a particular clinic. Patient support groups in your locality can probably put you in touch with people who have attended these clinics and may give invaluable help based on personal experience. For more on NHS and private treatment (including costs), see 'Assisted conception' on page 43.

WHAT TESTS WILL WE NEED?

The number of fertility tests that you will require generally depends on the complexity of your problem. It is impossible to generalise and cover all the possibilities. Outlined below are some common investigations that provide a basic diagnosis for most couples.

Blood tests

You will need to have a test to assess your rubella (German measles) status. German measles is a fairly mild illness in women, causing a slight rash, swollen glands and aching joints, but it can damage an unborn baby if it is caught during early pregnancy. If you are not immune, you will be offered an immunisation. You should avoid pregnancy for four weeks afterwards, which is when the test should be repeated to confirm that the immunisation has been effective.

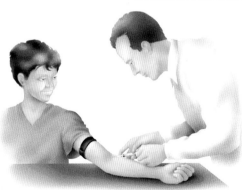

Some blood samples will be taken to assess your general health and other specific factors.

A full blood count will assess your overall health and will make sure that you are not suffering from anaemia. Additional blood tests will be needed to check your hormone levels and some of these samples will need to be taken at specific times in the woman's monthly cycle. Follicle-stimulating hormone (FSH) and luteinising hormone (LH) levels are usually measured at the end of the woman's period and give an indication of the reserve supply and quality of the eggs that are ripening in her ovaries. Progesterone is measured about a week before her period is due, to assess whether a woman is ovulating (releasing eggs) normally. Thyroid hormone levels may also be measured. These control the rate at which the body's cells work (the metabolic rate). If a woman's thyroid gland is underactive, this can interfere with the quality of eggs that she releases and can also increase her risk of miscarriage.

You may also be tested for evidence of a previous infection with *Chlamydia*, which can damage or block a woman's fallopian tubes. If high levels of chlamydia antibodies are present, both partners will be treated with a suitable antibiotic. Treating a couple at this stage will not correct or prevent tubal damage that has already occurred, but it will prevent further reactivation of *Chlamydia*, which may occur during a laparoscopy or other pelvic surgery.

Ultrasound scans

At your first visit to a consultant, he or she may arrange for you to have an ultrasound scan of your pelvis. An ultrasound scan is painless and only Involves a short, outpatient

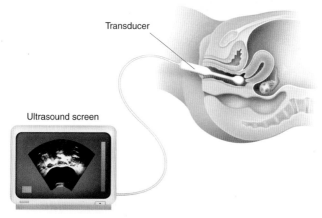

An ultrasound scan produces a photographic image using sound waves.

appointment. It produces an echo image using sound waves. As the waves bounce off different parts of your body, the echoes form a picture.

An ultrasound scan enables the consultant to assess the health of your ovaries and uterus, and to see how well your ovaries are working. It is possible to assess whether follicles are developing or whether there are any abnormalities, such as polycystic ovaries. In addition, your uterus is examined for the presence of a normal endometrial lining, which is appropriate for the stage of your monthly cycle, and any medical problems, such as fibroids (non-cancerous growths in the uterus) or developmental abnormalities. However, an ultrasound scan cannot diagnose conditions such as endometriosis (where tissue resembling the lining of the uterus is found in the pelvis) or blockages of the fallopian tubes.

In a few specialised centres, additional ultrasound techniques may be available. Studies of the developing follicle and blood flow around the ovaries (Doppler flow studies) are sometimes used to investigate infertility. Another technique called contrast ultrasound involves passing a fluid into the cavity of the uterus. The fluid is of a particular consistency so that it shows up clearly on ultrasound. Its flow along the fallopian tubes can be traced in this way, and any blockages revealed.

Hysterosalpingogram (HSG)

This is an X-ray picture to check whether the cavity of your uterus is normal and whether your fallopian tubes are open. It is often carried out in addition to a laparoscopy (see page 27) because it also gives information about the delicate lining

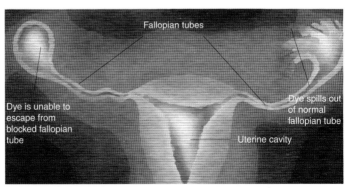

A hysterosalpingogram (HSG) involves passing dye, which shows up white on X-ray film, into the uterus and fallopian tubes. This gives information on any abnormalities.

inside the tubes. Passing a dye into the uterus, which shows up white on the X-ray films, gives information about any blockage or kinking of the tubes. It will also reveal whether there is a collection of fluid at the blockage (a hydrosalpinx). This procedure usually involves a short, outpatient appointment and is sometimes uncomfortable.

Laparoscopy

This is usually a day-case procedure under a general anaesthetic. It involves making a small cut in your abdomen, usually just under your navel so you won't have any noticeable scarring. A laparoscopy allows careful inspection of your ovaries, uterus and fallopian tubes, and can identify polycystic ovaries and uterine fibroids.

A blue-coloured dye is injected through the cervix and uterus, and can be clearly seen by the surgeon as it passes through your fallopian tubes and spills freely from the ends of the tubes if they are open and healthy. The blue dye is completely harmless and will be passed out in the woman's urine within a few hours. If your tubes are scarred or distorted, the tubal lining may be damaged. Further evidence for this may come from elevated antibody levels in the chlamydia blood test, which suggests that chlamydia infection is present. Adhesions (bands of scar tissue) and endo-metriosis may be distorting your fallopian tubes or ovaries; this is best treated by surgery. Medical

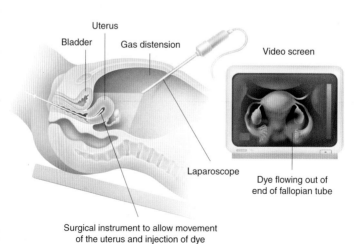

A laparoscopy allows careful inspection of the ovaries, uterus and fallopian tubes through a narrow 'telescope' with an attached video camera inserted into the abdomen.

treatment of endometriosis is of little value in improving the chance of pregnancy. For more on this, see 'Treating infertility' on page 33.

A hysteroscopy (direct examination of the interior of the uterus with a viewing instrument) may be advised at the same time as a laparoscopy to check the cavity of your uterus and the openings into the inner end of your fallopian tubes. This may allow any adhesions or polyps (growths) in the cavity of the uterus to be seen and, if necessary, removed.

Other tests

• **Seminal fluid analysis:** This is carried out on a sample of semen, which is examined under a microscope. The technician can count the number of sperm in a measured volume of semen. The sample is usually produced by masturbation. Generally, two to three days' abstinence from intercourse is recommended before the test. A diagnosis of a sperm problem should never be made from a single sperm sample. If the first test result shows low numbers or complete absence of sperm, it should be repeated.

Sperm analysis can also be used to assess the motility (swimming ability) of sperm and whether there are any abnormalities present (involving a count of the number of physically normal and abnormal sperm). Every man, even the most fertile, will still be producing some sperm that are non-motile or abnormally formed. Some men produce anti-sperm antibodies, which can cause the heads of the sperm (or occasionally the tails) to stick together, if they are present in seminal fluid. This reduces sperm motility and severely reduces the chance of fertilisation. Anti-sperm antibodies can also be produced by some women in their cervical mucus.

• **Postcoital testing (PCT):** This may be done if the sperm count appears to be normal and ovulation has been confirmed. It is occasionally undertaken instead of a seminal fluid analysis. It detects whether sperm survive normally within the woman's cervical mucus. Using a syringe, a sample of mucus is taken from the woman's cervix shortly before ovulation. The sample is taken about 12 hours after the couple have had intercourse, and is then examined immediately through a microscope. If more than three motile (moving) sperm are seen in each field of view under the microscope, this is termed a 'positive test'. If no sperm or no motile sperm are seen, this may indicate a problem with sperm function – either in their ability to penetrate the woman's mucus or in their survival capacity. A woman's cervical mucus could also be abnormal, containing antibodies against sperm.

WHAT MAY THE TESTS SHOW?

The most common causes of infertility in women are ovulation failure and blockage or damage of the fallopian tubes. Ovulation failure may be evident from infrequent or absent menstrual periods. However, in some women, it will be diagnosed only by means of a blood test to measure their levels of progesterone. Endometriosis and cervical mucus disorders are less frequent causes. It is not certain that endometriosis causes infertility – it may be present only because it is more common in women who have not been pregnant for some time. In men, poor sperm function or a very low sperm count is more common

TESTING FOR COMMON INFERTILITY PROBLEMS

Problem	Summary of problem	Common tests
Chlamydia infection	Damages or blocks fallopian tubes	Blood test HSG
Polycystic ovaries	Affect ovulation or egg quality	Ultrasound Blood tests Laparoscopy
Fibroids	Growths in uterus; block fallopian tubes	Ultrasound Laparoscopy
Problem with endometrial lining	Fertilised egg may not implant	Ultrasound Hysteroscopy
Blockage of fallopian tubes	Prevents fertilisation	Laparoscopy HSG
Adhesions	Build up of scar tissue interferes with ovulation	Laparoscopy
Endometriosis	Formation of adhesions	Laparoscopy
Reduced or no sperm production or sperm abnormalities	Prevents fertilisation	Seminal fluid analysis
Cervical mucus	Sperm cannot survive in mucus	Postcoital test

Test	Reason to undertake this test
FSH	Examines the ability of the ovary to produce follicles, assesses the reserve supply of eggs and with LH levels predicts polycystic ovary syndrome
LH	With FSH levels predicts polycystic ovary syndrom
Progesterone	Determines if ovulation took place
TSH	Detects a poorly functioning thyroid gland which can affect fertility
Prolactin	A hormone which, if overproduced, suppresses ovulation and menstruation
Semen analysis	Checks for the presence and quantity of sperm
Postcoital test	Checks the function of sperm, and the quality of cervical mucus

FSH, follicle-stimulating hormone; IU/l, international unit per litre; LH, luteinis

than a complete failure of sperm production. In about 15 per cent of cases, subfertility has more than one cause.

In almost a third of couples, the results of all their investigations will be normal. This situation is called unexplained infertility, and is frustrating for couples who want to know why they can't conceive. In many cases, there will not be a problem at all and the couple will simply have been unlucky. In others, subtle or minor factors will be impairing their fertility, but their chance of achieving a pregnancy will still be realistic without resorting to active, and possibly

...onditions required for the test	Normal values and units
...est in the first week of the woman's ...ycle	1–9 IU/l
...s for FSH	1–9 IU/l
...est done 5–10 days before a ...eriod is due	> 30 nmol/l
...ny time or day	0.3–3.0 IU/l
...ny time or day	100–800 nmol/l
...xamined within 1 hour of production ...sample	Count > 20 million sperm/ml Normality > 30 per cent Motility > 50 per cent
...amined within 8–12 hours of ...tercourse at midcycle ...ucus stretching to at least 10 cm ...H 6–8.5	Normal: > 3 motile sperm Impaired: 1–3 sperm Negative: 0 sperm All per high-power microsope field (× 400 magnification)

...mone; TSH, thyroid-stimulating hormone.

stressful, intrusive or expensive, treatments.

Couples with unexplained infertility who have been trying for a pregnancy for more than three years, or where the woman is over 35 years of age, need to consider active fertility treatments. There are a number of options. Ovulation induction may improve their chance of pregnancy by stimulating the release of more than one egg each month. Intrauterine insemination in combination with ovulation induction may give a higher chance of pregnancy (15 to 20 per cent per cycle). In vitro fertilisation (IVF) or gamete intrafallopian transfer (GIFT)

THE COMMON CAUSES OF INFERTILITY

Cause	Percentage
Women	
Ovulation failure	20
Fallopian tube damage	15
Scarring from endometriosis	6
Cervical mucus problems	3
Men	
Poor sperm function/low sperm count	25
Failure of sperm production/release	2
Both partners	
Unexplained infertility	28
Problems with intercourse	6
Miscellaneous other causes	11
	——
	116

The total adds up to more than 100 per cent because 16 per cent of couples have more than one cause for their infertility.

treatments offer the best chance of pregnancy, equivalent or better than the chance of natural conception for normal fertile couples. However, they also involve the greatest commitment and expense for the couple concerned. For more on these treatments, see 'Treating infertility'.

KEY POINTS

✓ Most couples should wait a year before seeking help if they are experiencing difficulty in conceiving

✓ Couples should have the full range of investigations for a complete and accurate diagnosis

Treating infertility

Most infertility problems don't require assisted conception techniques, such as in vitro fertilisation (IVF), but can be treated with simpler methods. The treatments you will be offered will depend on the cause of your infertility. If you are not ovulating properly, you may be offered either medication to correct the cause or fertility drugs to stimulate the ovaries.

If you have blocked or damaged fallopian tubes, you may need surgery, either as an open operation or, increasingly, by laparoscopy ('keyhole' surgery). Disorders of sperm function respond poorly to drug treatment. Instead, you may be offered sperm donation or assisted conception (for more details, see later sections). Drug treatment for endometriosis does not appear to improve fertility.

OVULATION INDUCTION

If you are not ovulating or do so irregularly, your chances of con-ceiving are obviously diminished. There are several causes of ovulation failure, and most cause either a complete absence of menstrual periods (amenorrhoea) or infrequent periods (oligo-menorrhoea). Provided you have not gone through an early meno-pause, the available treatments are generally very effective.

Some conditions that may require more complex medical treatment or, occasionally, even surgical treatment include: hypo-pituitarism (underactivity of the pituitary gland, which leads to less follicle-stimulating hormone (FSH) and luteinising hormone (LH) being produced); hypogonadotrophic hypogonadism (poor ovarian activity caused by inadequate stimulation of the pituitary gland); hyperprolactinaemia (excessive prolactin hormone production by a small benign (non-cancerous) tumour of the pituitary gland) and polycystic ovarian syndrome (where the hormone signals to the ovaries are unbalanced, leading to development of multiple small cysts).

If your periods have stopped because of excessive or sudden weight loss, you may respond to dietary measures alone, but most other causes of ovulation failure are likely to require specific hormone treatments. The methods used to induce ovulation include clomiphene citrate, bromocriptine, pulsed GnRH, gonadotrophin therapy and ovarian diathermy.

Women with ovulation failure caused by a premature menopause will not respond to ovulation induction treatments. However, their problem can be bypassed by using donated eggs for IVF or GIFT. For more details of these treatments, see 'Assisted conception' on page 43.

OVULATION INDUCTION USING HORMONE TREATMENTS

Clomiphene citrate
Clomiphene citrate tablets are used to stop a woman's own oestrogen hormones from reducing the production of FSH and LH in her pituitary gland. They are effective therefore only in women who are already producing oestrogen, mainly those with polycystic ovarian syndrome. The tablets are taken for five days in the early part of the menstrual cycle.

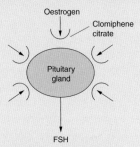

For the first five days of the menstrual cycle, clomiphene citrate blocks oestrogen from inhibiting FSH production by the pituitary gland

Bromocriptine
Bromocriptine tablets are taken daily to reduce prolactin levels. They are used for women who are producing excessive amounts of prolactin hormone, which is blocking their normal production of FSH and LH.

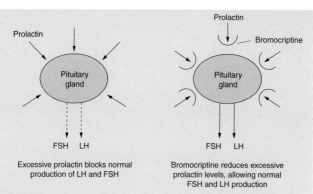

Excessive prolactin blocks normal production of LH and FSH

Bromocriptine reduces excessive prolactin levels, allowing normal FSH and LH production

Pulsed GnRH

GnRH stimulates the pituitary gland to release the hormones FSH and LH, which then stimulate the woman's ovaries to develop and release eggs. It is used in women who are not producing sufficient GnRH to stimulate their pituitary gland. GnRH is given by a small portable battery-controlled syringe pump through a fine tube and needle, usually inserted under the skin, but occasionally into a vein. Small doses of GnRH are injected by the miniature pump every 90 minutes over the course of two to three weeks.

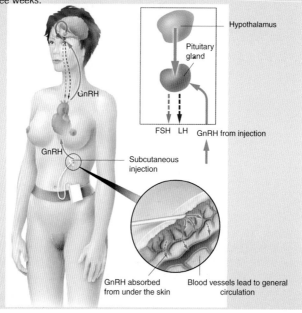

GnRH absorbed from under the skin

Blood vessels lead to general circulation

Gonadotrophins

Gonadotrophin injections contain FSH or a mixture of FSH and LH. They stimulate the ovaries directly, and are used either when a woman's own pituitary gland is unable to produce FSH and LH (perhaps because of previous pituitary surgery) or when treatment by pulsed gonadotrophin-releasing hormone (GnRH) or clomiphene citrate has not been successful in inducing ovulation. The gonadotrophins are given by daily injections, usually for about 10 to 15 days. The lowest dose is used initially and increased only if the woman's ovaries are not responding.

The aim of the treatment is to produce one or two mature follicles and then to induce ovulation with a single injection of a different drug (human chorionic gonadotrophin or hCG). The couple are advised to have intercourse at this time because ovulation will occur about 40 hours after the hCG injection. For women who have ovulation induction with gonadotrophin drugs, there is a 15 to 20 per cent chance of conception in each cycle and about a 60 per cent chance after six cycles.

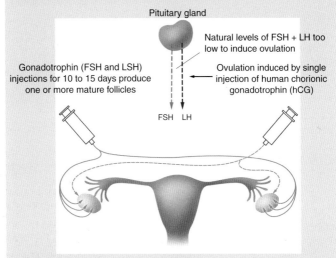

Pituitary gland

Natural levels of FSH + LH too low to induce ovulation

Gonadotrophin (FSH and LSH) injections for 10 to 15 days produce one or more mature follicles

Ovulation induced by single injection of human chorionic gonadotrophin (hCG)

FSH   LH

Gonadotrophins are powerful hormones and can cause multiple pregnancy and ovarian hyperstimulation syndrome (for more details, see 'Assisted conception' on page 43). Therefore, the woman requires careful monitoring by the fertility clinic every two to three days. The follicle size and number are measured by ultrasound, and follicle hormone production is measured by blood oestrogen tests.

Some women having gonadotrophin treatment will be asked to take an additional drug called a GnRH analogue (GnRHa). This prevents their own body hormones from interfering and triggering the release of their eggs prematurely. The GnRHa is usually given as a nasal spray several times daily from about two weeks before the gonadotrophin injections up to the time of the single injection of hCG

Ovarian diathermy
Ovarian diathermy (electric cautery) is used to treat infertility caused by polycystic ovarian syndrome. It is thought to work by destroying some of the dense tissue in the centre of the ovaries. At the time of a laparoscopy, under general anaesthetic, a needle is pushed into the deeper, dense part of the ovary and several pulses of electric current destroy some of this tissue. This reduces the abnormal balance of hormones produced by the ovaries, which in turn reduces the raised level of LH.

This procedure can be useful for women who are not responding to clomiphene and whose LH concentrations are raised (the persistently high LH levels interfere with normal follicular development). Ovarian diathermy brings about ovulation in up to 50 per cent of women who are treated and pregnancy in 15 to 20 per cent. The effect is temporary, lasting about six to nine months.

The risk of ovarian cancer
There are concerns about whether the use of clomiphene or gonadotrophins may lead to increased risks of ovarian cancer later in life. These risks are difficult to quantify, partly because women with ovulation failure may have a slightly increased risk of ovarian cancer anyway, but also because a pregnancy from any successful treatment greatly reduces the risk of ovarian cancer.

The evidence available at present does not suggest that these treatments increase the risk of ovarian cancer when used appropriately.

TUBAL SURGERY
If your fallopian tubes are blocked, surgery may be necessary. Blocked fallopian tubes are often caused by an infection, usually from *Chlamydia*. If an infection damages the delicate lining inside the tubes, this cannot be corrected and the fallopian tubes may not be able to function normally. Sometimes, tubal surgery is indicated because of damage from endometriosis or

because of scar tissue (adhesions) from previous surgery.

The tubes may be unblocked by open surgery under general anaesthesia using special microscopic techniques. Increasingly, these types of operations are being done through the laparoscope (keyhole surgery), sometimes at the time of diagnosis.

The success of surgery

The success of the surgery depends on the severity of the tubal disease. With only minor adhesions, about 70 to 80 per cent of women may conceive within 12 months. With more severe disease or tubal blockage, this may fall to only 25 to 30 per cent and, if an infection has caused the damage, the success rate may be as low as 10 per cent after 12 months.

Although surgery for more extensive tubal damage might increase a couple's chance of success, it will usually still be unrealistically low. In this situation, IVF offers a much greater chance of pregnancy. However, if a woman's tubes have been blocked and have swollen up with accumulated fluid secretions (a hydrosalpinx), this can reduce the chance of conception

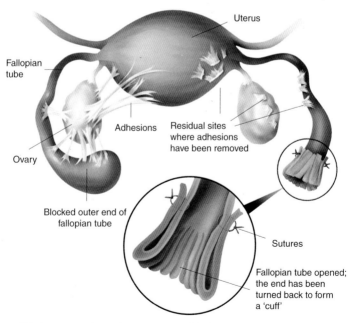

Uterus

Fallopian tube

Adhesions

Residual sites where adhesions have been removed

Ovary

Blocked outer end of fallopian tube

Sutures

Fallopian tube opened; the end has been turned back to form a 'cuff'

Tubal surgery can be used to correct some of the blockages that can occur in the fallopian tubes.

even with IVF. Surgery may then be advised to remove her fallopian tubes before any IVF treatment.

If the woman has severely damaged fallopian tubes, but the couple cannot afford IVF, she may still wish to consider surgery. Surgery may seem inappropriate because it hardly improves the chance of pregnancy. However, when there is no other way of achieving a pregnancy, even a very small chance of conception may be better than no chance.

Possible risks

If a woman conceives after tubal surgery, there is a 10 to 15 per cent chance that the pregnancy will implant in one of her fallopian tubes (an ectopic pregnancy) rather than in the cavity of her uterus. This is a potentially serious condition that requires emergency surgery.

TREATING SPERM DISORDERS

Sperm disorders are the most common cause of subfertility. Hormone treatments and artificial insemination using the husband's sperm (AIH) are not effective, apart from in very rare circumstances. IVF may be appropriate for treating minor disorders of sperm function, but in most cases ICSI (intracytoplasmic sperm injection) offers the best chance of pregnancy.

ICSI (intracytoplasmic sperm injection)

In most fertility clinics, the chance of

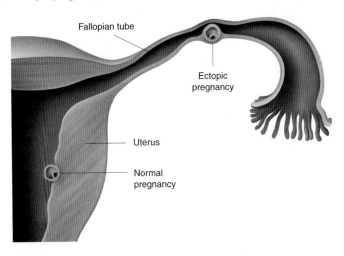

An ectopic pregnancy is a potentially serious condition, in which the fertilised egg is implanted in the wall of the fallopian tube, and not the uterus.

pregnancy per ICSI treatment cycle varies from 12 to 30 per cent (average about 18 per cent) with live birth rates of 10 to 25 per cent (average about 15 per cent). These figures are only a few per cent lower than the results from standard IVF in couples where the man has normal sperm function.

Even for men who are not producing any sperm in their ejaculate, ICSI offers an increased chance of pregnancy if sperm can be collected surgically from the epididymes or testes. For more details about ICSI, see 'Assisted conception' on page 43.

Sperm donation

If the man's sperm counts are consistently low or abnormal, or he is not producing any sperm at all, the use of donor sperm may be suggested. Donor sperm may also be advised when there is a risk that a man may pass on a serious genetic disease to his children through his own sperm. Pregnancy rates are generally seven to ten per cent per cycle. The rate of conception is lower than for normal fertile couples, mainly because only freeze–stored donor sperm are used and the freezing and thawing of sperm reduces their fertilising potential.

For more on sperm donation, see 'Egg or sperm donation' on page 62.

TREATMENT FOR ENDOMETRIOSIS

Endometriosis occurs when cells from the lining of the uterus are found in other places in the abdominal cavity. These cells respond to hormonal changes throughout the menstrual cycle, causing bleeding during the menstrual period. As the cells are now in an enclosed space, the blood cannot escape, as would be the case in the uterus where blood drains through the cervix. The inflammation that endometriosis causes can lead to severe abdominal pain, pelvic tenderness and painful sexual intercourse. Scarring may also occur, forming adhesions (bands of scar tissue), which can distort or block the fallopian tubes or prevent eggs passing from the ovaries to the fallopian tubes.

TREATMENT OPTIONS

There are various drug treatments for endometriosis, usually given for several months. These may reduce endometriosis symptoms, particularly the pain. However, all the effective drug treatments have contraceptive properties while they are being taken and there is no evidence that fertility is improved after treatment.

The whole area of effective treatment for infertile women with endometriosis is a matter of some debate. Although women with

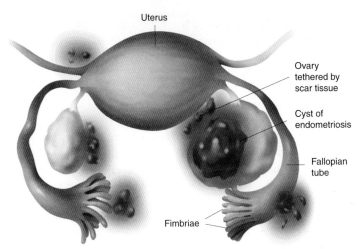

Although the fallopian tubes are open, and the delicate fimbriae at their outer ends are intact, scar tissue from previous bouts of endometriosis is limiting the normal mobility of the fallopian tubes, preventing them reaching the surface of the ovary to collect ripe eggs as they are released.

endometriosis may have a reduced chance of conceiving, current evidence shows that no drug or hormone therapy improves fertility.

If minor endometriosis is diagnosed by a laparoscopy, electrical cautery or laser can be used to destroy the deposits of endometriosis. This may improve fertility in some cases. More major disease requires open surgery that is often extensive. Diathermy or laser treatment may improve pregnancy rates by 30 per cent or more after surgery. For some women with endometriosis, IVF will offer their best chance of pregnancy.

KEY POINTS

✓ Not all fertility problems require IVF or other assisted conception treatments

✓ 'Simple' treatments are effective in the management of many cases of infertility

✓ Precise and accurate diagnosis is important to decide which treatments are most likely to be successful for each couple

Assisted conception

If simpler infertility treatments are unsuccessful or inappropriate, your doctor may suggest that you consider some form of assisted conception. These techniques won't treat the cause of your infertility, but will bypass it to increase your chance of conceiving. They include in vitro fertilisation (IVF), which is the original 'test tube baby' treatment, gamete intrafallopian transfer (GIFT), intrauterine insemination (IUI) and intracytoplasmic sperm injection (ICSI).

STAGES OF TREATMENT

Assisted conception involves several similar procedures. The first is the stimulation of the woman's ovaries to develop a number of

WHICH TREATMENT FOR WHICH PROBLEM?

Problem	Assisted conception technique
Fallopian tube damage	IVF
Unexplained infertility	GIFT, IUI or IVF
Endometriosis-related infertility	GIFT, IUI or IVF
Minor male infertility	IVF
Severe male infertility	ICSI
Absence of sperm	SSR and ICSI

IVF, in vitro fertilisation; GIFT, gamete intrafallopian transfer;
IUI, intrauterine insemination; ICSI, intracytoplasmic sperm injection;
SSR, surgical sperm recovery.

eggs using high doses of fertility hormone injections. This is referred to as superovulation. The second is the monitoring of the development of the woman's eggs by ultrasound scans and, in some clinics, measuring the oestrogen levels in her blood to know when the eggs are mature and ready to be fertilised. The third is the collection of sperm. These stages of treatment are all arranged as an outpatient. For IVF, GIFT and ICSI, the woman will need to be admitted to hospital as a day-case for collection of her eggs. For surgical sperm recovery, the man will usually be admitted as a day-case.

Superovulation

Several hormones are used to stimulate the woman's ovaries to produce additional mature eggs. In the first stage of treatment, her own hormones will be suppressed temporarily using a drug called a gonadotrophin-releasing hormone analogue (GnRHa). This is usually started about seven to ten days before she is due to start her period, in the cycle before assisted conception is planned.

The GnRHa is usually given as a nasal spray or a daily or monthly injection, and the woman will need to continue taking this until shortly before her eggs are mature. In some clinics, she may be given a seven-day course of progestogen tablets as well, to make sure that she sheds the lining of her uterus completely when she has her period.

Daily injections of human menopausal gonadotrophin (hMG), or a similar hormone preparation, are used to stimulate the development of follicles in the ovaries. The developing follicles are monitored as they mature by several ultrasound scans. In some clinics, blood samples are taken to monitor the levels of oestrogen produced by the ovaries.

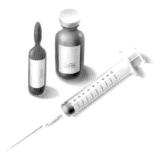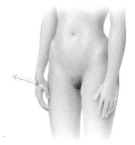

Superovulation involves the stimulation of the woman's ovaries to develop a number of eggs by injecting high doses of fertility hormones.

When the follicles are mature, a single injection of human chorionic gonadotrophin (hCG) is given to trigger the final stages of egg development and ovulation about 38 to 42 hours later. Once the hCG injection has been given, the woman stops using the GnRHa. However, because the GnRHa has been suppressing her own hormones, she will need some additional treatment to keep the lining of her uterus stable and receptive for a pregnancy over the following eight to ten days. This may be with one or two lower-dose hCG injections or with progestogen hormone injections or vaginal pessaries.

Sperm collection

The man will be asked to produce a semen sample early on the day of the woman's egg collection or ovulation. This may be into a pot containing culture fluid, or into two pots (a 'split' ejaculate), depending on the assessment of previous

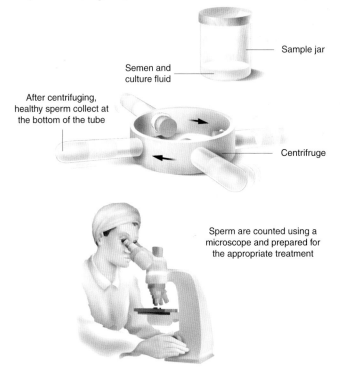

Sample jar

Semen and culture fluid

After centrifuging, healthy sperm collect at the bottom of the tube

Centrifruge

Sperm are counted using a microscope and prepared for the appropriate treatment

The man will be asked to prepare a semen sample early on the day of the woman's egg collection or ovulation.

semen samples. The semen is left for a short time to liquefy and then forced through some filtration fluid at high speed (a process called centrifugation). Any debris and abnormal sperm are separated out and healthy, intact sperm collect at the bottom. These are transferred to a test tube of fresh culture fluid. The number of sperm are counted and prepared for the appropriate treatment.

SSR

If the man is releasing no sperm in his ejaculate (azoospermia), surgical sperm recovery (SSR) techniques may be necessary. For men with obstructive azoospermia (where the tubes taking sperm from the testes are blocked), sperm may be collected by passing a needle through the skin of the scrotum into the testis itself, or into the coiled tubules on the surface of the testis, the epididymis. The sperm may be collected on the day the woman's eggs are collected or one or two days beforehand. Any extra sperm collected may be frozen and stored for future use to avoid the need for repeated SSR.

If the tubes are not blocked (non-obstructive azoospermia), the inside of the testis is thoroughly examined. This can be done as a day-case procedure under general anaesthetic. Several matchhead-sized pieces of tissue may be removed for examination under a microscope, as sperm production may be occurring only in small areas. The chance of collecting sperm is lower for men with non-obstructive azoospermia (50 to 60 per cent) than for men with obstructive azoospermia (about 95 per cent).

After SSR, the man will be advised to wear a firm support for 48 hours, and may need to take some simple pain-killers, such as aspirin or paracetamol. If SSR has been done as an open operation, he may need to rest for three to five days before returning to work.

BASICS OF THE TECHNIQUES

IUI (intrauterine insemination)

IUI is only suitable if the woman has healthy fallopian tubes, for example, if there is unexplained infertility or endometriosis-associated infertility. It raises the chance of pregnancy by increasing the number of eggs and sperm coming into contact with each other in the fallopian tubes. Occasionally, it may be used for minor degrees of male infertility, for women with impaired cervical mucus production or quality, and for rare situations where normal sexual intercourse is not possible.

The prepared sperm are concentrated into a small volume of culture fluid, less than a quarter of a

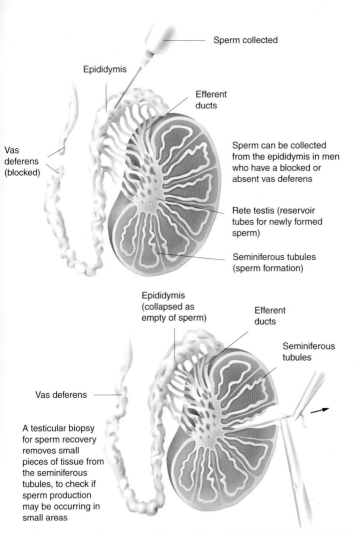

Sperm collected

Epididymis

Efferent ducts

Vas deferens (blocked)

Sperm can be collected from the epididymis in men who have a blocked or absent vas deferens

Rete testis (reservoir tubes for newly formed sperm)

Seminiferous tubules (sperm formation)

Epididymis (collapsed as empty of sperm)

Efferent ducts

Seminiferous tubules

Vas deferens

A testicular biopsy for sperm recovery removes small pieces of tissue from the seminiferous tubules, to check if sperm production may be occurring in small areas

If the man is releasing no sperm in his ejaculate, surgical sperm recovery techniques may be necessary.

teaspoonful. The procedure should not be painful, and no sedation or anaesthetic is required. An instrument called a speculum is inserted into the woman's vagina to allow a clear view of her cervix. The sperm are drawn up into a long, soft, narrow plastic tube with a syringe. The plastic tube is gently passed through the cervix to the top of her

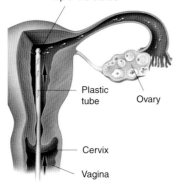

Sperm injected at top of the uterus

Plastic tube

Ovary

Cervix

Vagina

IUI (intrauterine insemination).

uterus where the sperm are released. The plastic tube is slowly withdrawn and, after a few minutes' rest, to allow the woman's cervical mucus to seal off the passage through her cervix, the woman can get up and return home.

Egg collection

For GIFT, IVF or ICSI, the woman's eggs are collected just before they are ready to be ovulated, usually about 32 to 36 hours after she has had her single injection of hCG. Most egg collection procedures are done through the woman's vagina using an ultrasound scanner to guide a needle into each of the follicles and draw off the fluid and eggs. The needle passes down a hollow guide tube, which is clipped to the side of the ultrasound probe, and through the top of her vagina into her ovaries. The egg collection

is carried out as a day-case procedure under sedation or a light general anaes-thetic, and usually takes about 20 to 40 minutes. As each follicle is drained, the test tube of fluid collected is passed to an embryologist, who examines it under a microscope to identify the egg. The eggs are transferred to carefully labelled tubes containing nutrient-rich culture fluid and placed in an incubator.

Occasionally, the eggs will be collected at a laparoscopy operation under general anaesthetic. The laparoscope is a narrow telescope-like instrument that is inserted through a 'keyhole' incision at the woman's navel. A needle is passed through the abdominal wall to collect the eggs under the direct vision of the surgeon through the laparoscope. This technique is more commonly used when a couple are having GIFT treatment, because the woman then needs a laparoscopy anyway to place up to three eggs and the prepared sperm in her fallopian tubes.

GIFT (gamete intrafallopian transfer)

GIFT is suitable for the same infertility problems as IUI. The woman's eggs are collected from her ovaries, and up to three mature eggs are transferred back to her fallopian tubes. If her eggs have been collected via her vagina, she is

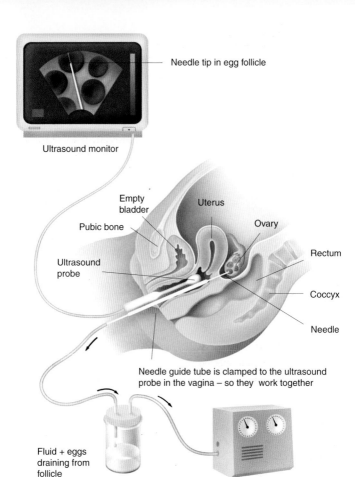

Needle tip in egg follicle

Ultrasound monitor

Empty bladder

Uterus

Pubic bone

Ovary

Ultrasound probe

Rectum

Coccyx

Needle

Needle guide tube is clamped to the ultrasound probe in the vagina – so they work together

Fluid + eggs draining from follicle

Suction pump

For most GIFT, IVF and ICSI techniques, the woman's eggs are collected through the vagina using an ultrasound scanner to guide a needle into the follicles and draw off the fluid and eggs.

given a full general anaesthetic for a laparoscopy. With the laparoscope in place, the outer end of a fallopian tube is lifted up with special forceps. A narrow, rigid metal tube is passed through her abdominal wall and carefully threaded into the outer end of her fallopian tube for about two centimetres.

At the same time, the sperm and eggs are prepared under the microscope. A small drop of fluid containing about 20,000 sperm is drawn into the fine, soft, plastic GIFT

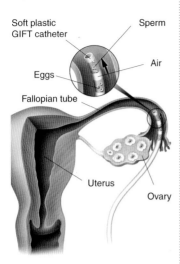

Soft plastic GIFT catheter

Sperm

Air

Eggs

Fallopian tube

Uterus

Ovary

GIFT (gamete intrafallopian transfer).

catheter, followed by a small pocket of air, a small drop of fluid containing up to three eggs, another small pocket of air and a final drop of fluid containing about 20,000 sperm. The GIFT catheter is threaded down the rigid metal tube into one of the woman's fallopian tubes and the sperm and eggs are released to mix together.

IVF (in vitro fertilisation)
IVF is suitable for women with damaged fallopian tubes. About one to six hours after egg collection, 50,000 to 200,000 sperm are added to the small quantity of culture fluid around each egg. This mixture is then transferred to an incubator.

The eggs are inspected under a microscope 18 to 24 hours later. If

fertilisation has occurred, the early embryos (called zygotes) are transferred to fresh culture fluid and then returned to the incubator for 24 to 48 hours to allow them to develop further. The most mature embryos, up to a maximum of three, are selected for transfer back to the woman's uterus. Any additional embryos can be freeze-stored for later use if they are of sufficiently good quality.

The embryo transfer procedure is virtually identical to intrauterine insemination. However, a slightly narrower catheter is used and the embryos are transferred in a much smaller volume of culture fluid – literally a tiny drop. The woman's cervix is viewed with a speculum. The embryo transfer catheter is carefully passed through the cervix to the upper end of the uterus where the embryos are injected. The catheter is then gently withdrawn and checked under a microscope to confirm that the embryos have been released. After a couple of minutes' rest, the woman can get up and return home.

ICSI (intracytoplasmic sperm injection)
ICSI is used when there is severe male factor infertility. This may be the result of a very low sperm count or severely impaired sperm function. It is also necessary when

sperm have been collected surgically, because the number of sperm will be low and their swimming ability reduced. ICSI may also be advised for some couples who have had failed fertilisation with previous standard IVF treatment.

ICSI involves the direct injection of a selected individual sperm into each egg in the laboratory under a high-power microscope. It is appropriate only for completely mature eggs. An individual sperm is selected from the man's sample. It is immobilised (usually by fracturing its tail) so that it can't swim back out of the egg after it has been injected. The sperm is then carefully loaded backwards into an ultra-fine glass injection needle.

Under the microscope, the egg is held firmly in position by suction onto the end of a thin, blunt, glass tube. The glass needle containing the single sperm approaches the egg slowly until it has pierced and entered the nucleus of the egg. The sperm is then injected. Even with an experienced embryologist, about one in 20 eggs will be damaged by the injection procedure. About 50 to 65 per cent of the mature eggs injected will fertilise after ICSI.

Possible complications

Complications are uncommon with assisted conception techniques. However, sometimes the treatment is discontinued because the woman's ovaries respond excessively or inadequately to hormone stimulation. The hormone treatment can sometimes cause side effects (such as headaches with GnRHa, or tenderness and localised redness at the site of the daily hMG injections). Other potential problems are that fewer eggs are collected than expected, there may be slight

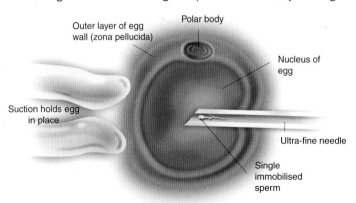

Outer layer of egg wall (zona pellucida)

Polar body

Nucleus of egg

Suction holds egg in place

Ultra-fine needle

Single immobilised sperm

ICSI (intracytoplasmic sperm injection).

vaginal bleeding after egg collection, the eggs do not fertilise at IVF or there are technical difficulties with embryo transfer (which may then require a short general anaesthetic).

Two major complications are ovarian hyperstimulation syndrome and multiple pregnancy. Ovarian hyperstimulation syndrome (OHSS) occurs when the woman's ovaries enlarge with fluid-filled cysts. It occurs in about three to five per cent of IVF treatments and is a complication that occurs only after embryos have been transferred back to the woman's uterus. It is more common if the woman's ovaries have responded particularly well to hormone stimulation or if she has polycystic ovarian syndrome. Mild symptoms include lower abdominal discomfort, bloating and nausea. More severe – and rarer – symptoms include abdominal swelling and pain, vomiting, nausea, shortness of breath (particularly when lying down) and reduced urine production.

A multiple pregnancy (twins, triplets or more) is more likely with assisted conception, as up to a maximum of three eggs or embryos are returned to the fallopian tubes. About a third of the multiple births in the UK are now thought to result from assisted conception treatments. The risk of multiple pregnancy will vary depending on the individual clinic and the couple's circumstances (particularly the woman's age and whether she has had previous pregnancies). As a rough guide, about 65 to 75 per cent of pregnancies will be singleton, 20 to 30 per cent twins and three to five per cent triplets. Multiple pregnancies carry an increased risk of complications for the mother and babies, and increased emotional and financial pressures for the couple. To minimise the risk of multiple pregnancy – particularly triplets – some couples decide to have only two eggs or embryos transferred during GIFT or IVF treatment.

TREATMENTS THROUGH THE NHS

The extent of NHS funding for assisted conception treatments varies in different parts of the UK. The range and extent of treatments available may also change from year to year, and you should ask your GP for advice. You may also get useful information from the local branch of one of the national patient support groups, whose addresses are given at the end of this book.

There may be restrictions on couples who are eligible for NHS treatment, often based on the woman's age, the type of fertility problem and whether the couple already have a child. If treatment is available, there is likely to be a waiting list, varying from several months to two or three years. The simpler and cheaper (although also less successful) treatments, such as IUI, may be more readily available.

THE COST OF PRIVATE TREATMENT

Treatment costs vary between fertility clinics. Most clinics charge separately for an initial consultation and any preliminary investigations. However, your GP may be willing to organise some of these initial tests. If you have private health insurance, this may cover the cost of your initial consultation and assessment (although not your treatment), as this is essentially an investigation of whether assisted conception is appropriate.

Most clinics do not include drug and hormone costs in their treatment charges, as the dosages needed will vary for different women. These are usually paid separately. In some cases, your family doctor may be prepared to prescribe the necessary drugs, even if only for the first cycle of treatment.

APPROXIMATE COSTS OF FERTILITY TREATMENTS

Initial consultation	£80–150
Specific initial investigations (in addition to general infertility tests)	£100–200
Drugs (complete package)[a]	£350–1,500
IUI	£600–1,200
IVF or GIFT	£1,400–2,400
ICSI	£2,000–3,400
SSR[b]	£350–1,000
Freezing and storage of sperm or embryos (five years)	£120–400
Freeze–stored embryo transfer	£150–300

[a]This is in addition to any assisted conception treatment. The lower cost would be for a young woman with responsive ovaries having IUI. The higher cost would be for a woman over 40 having IVF or GIFT.

[b]This is in addition to ICSI treatment. The variation in cost depends on whether local or general anaesthetic is used and whether or not exploration of the testes is needed.

KEY POINTS

✓ Assisted conception offers the best chance of pregnancy for about 50 per cent of infertile couples

✓ ICSI treatment can be used to overcome severe male infertility

✓ Most men who are not producing any sperm in their ejaculate can have their sperm collected surgically

✓ There are only limited provisions for assisted conception treatments within the NHS

Case studies

The case studies below are designed to illustrate in practice how some of the investigations mentioned already are interpreted and applied in selecting appropriate treatments. They should be read as the narrative on the left column and the explanation on the right.

CASE STUDY 1: OVULATION FAILURE

Case history

Jane is 26. She has been married for three years. For contraception, she has used an oral contraceptive (the Pill) since she was 20, until two years ago. She and her husband then decided they wanted to start a family. Since coming off the Pill, her periods have become quite irregular and unpredictable, and sometimes she has not had one for two to three months. She is happily married and has a steady job that she likes, although it is occasionally stressful. Almost two years have passed without getting pregnant, so she asked her GP to refer her to see a specialist.

While awaiting an appointment

Comments, investigations and management outlines

Stressful situations can cause cycle irregularities. These usually need to be fairly profound, e.g. recent bereavement, moving countries or beginning a new job.

- *First tests: early follicular phase tests are follicle-stimulating hormone (FSH) and luteinising hormone (LH)*
- *Other tests of value are those for thyroid-stimulating hormone (TSH) and prolactin*
- *Her results were: FSH: 4.5 IU/l (normal) (IU = international unit, a measure of the hormone)*

to see a specialist, Jane's GP did some blood tests; the first in the early part of her menstrual cycle and the second about 5 to 10 days before her next period was due. These showed absence of ovulation so her GP prescribed a mild ovulation-stimulating agent, clomiphene citrate. Despite taking this for three months, there was no sign of ovulation.

When the specialist saw her, an ultrasound scan of her ovaries was done. This showed an appearance of polycystic ovarian syndrome (PCOS), and was in agreement with the blood tests that had already been taken. In view of this and the failure to respond to mild ovulation induction, laparoscopy and ovarian diathermy were advised.

At laparoscopy, the ovaries were white and enlarged, the typical appearance of PCOS. Ovarian diathermy was undertaken. After the operation, LH levels dropped to normal. Spontaneous ovulation with regular cycles returned. Jane has not yet conceived but has had five ovulatory cycles since her treatment.

LH: 15.9 IU/l (raised) TSH and prolactin were normal

- *Second tests: The main test done at this time is progesterone: it was 4 nmol/l (reduced)*

These indicate failure of ovulation, which is most probably the result of polycystic ovarian syndrome (PCOS).

Ovarian diathermy is thought to work by destroying some of the stromal tissue in the ovary. This reduces the abnormal balance of hormones produced by the ovaries, which in turn reduces the raised level of LH.

After the operation, the blood LH level dropped from 15.9 to 3.4 IU/l. As expected, this more normal balance of hormone signals to the ovaries permitted the return of normal ovulation.

The effect is not permanent and evidence of PCOS on ultrasound scan and by blood tests will return, probably within a year.

CASE STUDY 2: TUBAL DAMAGE

Case history

Jean is 23, and has been living with her current boyfriend for 14 months. She was not concerned about getting pregnant when they

Comments, investigations and management outlines

Having several partners increases the risk of catching a sexually

started to live together and they have not used contraception. She has had several long relationships in the past with other men, and occasional one-night stands. Before meeting her current partner, she took the Pill as she didn't trust her partners enough to rely on them for contraception.

Over the past four years, she has had several episodes of lower abdominal pain, some of which were thought to be grumbling appendicitis and she was admitted to hospital during the last episode, as the pain was so severe.

To investigate the cause of the pain, she had some swabs taken from her cervix, and some blood tests and a laparoscopy were done. As a result of these, the diagnosis of an infection with *Chlamydia* was made, and an antibiotic was given to treat this.

The laparoscopy showed that both her tubes were blocked at their outer (fimbrial) ends (see the diagram on page 26). She was advised that she was unlikely to conceive and that surgery would be necessary when she wanted to try to get pregnant. This need not necessarily be done straightaway and, in fact, she was advised that she should delay this until she definitely wanted to conceive, as the best chance of success would be within the first year after surgery.

Her partner was advised of his

transmitted disease (STD). Although the Pill is effective in preventing unwanted pregnancy, it is not of any value in prevention of STDs and a condom is much more effective.

It is likely that these episodes of pain were in fact the result of Chlamydia. *Each episode of infection has about a 30 per cent chance of causing structural damage to the fallopian tubes.*

The swabs did not grow any bacteria – they often don't as Chlamydia *is particularly difficult to grow in the laboratory. The blood test looked at antibodies to chlamydia infection, both recent and past. These results were positive indicating considerable infection in the past and a current infection as well. An antibiotic such as ofloxacin or doxycycline is the recommended treatment and needs to be taken by both partners.*

Providing there is no further damage from another infection, the chances of success (getting pregnant within a year) from surgery are about 50 per cent. A hysterosalpingogram (HSG) would define the chance more accurately by giving information about the health of the inner tubal lining.

Surgery should not be done until the couple are sure that they want to proceed with a pregnancy.

need for antibiotic treatment as well. They were both advised that, as they might possibly have other sexually transmitted diseases (in addition to *Chlamydia*), they should visit the sexual health clinic. As yet, they have not decided to have any surgery.

The best chance of success is in the first year after surgery. If pregnancy hasn't occurred by then, it is unlikely to occur at all, usually because of damage to the delicate lining of the fallopian tubes. The first attempt at tubal surgery is the one most likely to be successful. Repeat attempts at surgery are generally not worthwhile.

CASE STUDY 3: MALE INFERTILITY

Case history

Mike is a fit 32-year-old man who exercises once or twice a week. He weighs 80 kilograms and doesn't smoke or drink alcohol. He has been married to Sue for three years, and they have been attempting to have a child for the last two years. They have decided to seek help through their GP.

His GP examined both of them, did a smear test for Sue and some blood tests, and a sperm sample examination was organised. Mike found producing the sample 'to order' a bit difficult but brought in his sample at the appointed time.

When the results returned, Sue's showed that she was ovulating with no other negative features. Mike's sperm sample seemed to suggest a problem as the sperm were clumping together. The GP felt that more specialist advice was necessary.

They were seen at the local

Comments, investigations and management outlines

Both smoking and drinking have been found to have detrimental effects on sperm quality, lowering their ability to fertilise eggs.

Mike's physical examination was normal. There were no hernias, and his testicles were normal in size and consistency.

The sperm sample result showed the following:

Volume	4 ml	Normal
Count	34 million/ml	Normal
Normality	55 per cent	Normal
Motility	20 per cent	Abnormal

(many sperm clumped together)

The postcoital test showed:

Normal cervical mucus quality and pH

Large numbers of sperm clumped together

Very few motile sperm seen

infertility clinic six months later. The specialist reviewed the results and suggested that the next step was a postcoital test. This was done a few weeks later and then they saw the specialist again to discuss the results.

Once again, the problem of sperm clumping together was found. The specialist suggested some additional tests on a sperm sample to check whether Mike was producing antibodies against his own sperm. When the results of these tests came back, they confirmed that anti-sperm antibodies were present in Mike's seminal fluid. The specialist told them that the likelihood of them conceiving on their own without help was low. He advised them to seek help from an assisted conception clinic, for IVF or perhaps for IUI. Mike and Sue were devastated at the thought of not being able to have a child without help. They have not decided what to do next.

The special sperm tests examined for anti-sperm antibodies. When these are present in seminal fluid, they cause the heads of the sperm (occasionally the tails) to stick together. This reduces sperm motility and severely reduces the chance of them reaching the outer ends of the women's fallopian tubes to fertilise an egg. Anti-sperm antibodies can also be produced by a woman in the mucus of her cervix. In Mike's case, they were present in the seminal fluid in high concentration and sperm clumping (agglutination) was severe.

Although some doctors have advocated the use of steroids to reduce the body's antibody response, the most effective way of achieving a pregnancy is to remove the sperm as quickly as possible from the seminal fluid, and inject the sperm into the uterus (IUI), or mix the sperm with eggs outside the body (IVF). If very high concentrations of antibody are present in the seminal fluid, ICSI is likely to offer the best chance of pregnancy.

CASE STUDY 4: UNEXPLAINED INFERTILITY

Case history

Janet and Peter have been married for five years, and stopped using contraception a year after they married when Janet was 29. As her

Comments, investigations and management outlines

Infertility does not run in families, although sperm disorders may be

sister had blocked tubes, they were concerned that any delay in diagnosis might make things more difficult for them. Two years ago, they asked to be referred by their GP to see a gynaecologist as Janet had not become pregnant. After six months of blood and sperm tests, an X-ray of Janet's uterus and a laparoscopy, they were told that there was no obvious cause for their failure to get pregnant. The gynaecologist was very positive and encouraging and said that, as this was the case, they had every chance of getting pregnant by themselves. The advice was they should relax, have regular intercourse and wait for it to happen.

The couple went on a holiday to Spain, and they went away for lots of weekends, but Janet didn't get pregnant. After a year, Janet suggested going back to see the gynaecologist. By then, they were becoming desperate. The gynaecologist went over things again, explained how everything was in good order and that no simple measures or treatment was going to help improve their chances. The only alternative to waiting for pregnancy to occur naturally was to intervene with IVF or GIFT.

After giving this some thought, and working out that they could afford two cycles of treatment, they

passed on and endometriosis is more commonly found in other family members than in the general population.

The diagnosis was essentially 'unexplained infertility' although this strictly requires three years of infertility. The role of factors such as stress is poorly understood, and difficult to define. Whenever formal studies of stress levels and stress chemicals have been done, no major differences are found in the infertile population. Yet there are many anecdotes of people who give up trying, adopt and then find themselves pregnant.

At the end of two years, 95 per cent of normal fertile couples will have conceived and, in the next year, there is still a likelihood of conception, though increasingly small (table on page 18). However, after three years, the chances of natural conception are very low and, realistically, the best chances then are from treatments such as IVF or GIFT.

Many IVF clinics will want to repeat some or all of the tests that are relevant. This is partly to have accurate results, partly to ensure nothing dramatic has changed since initial testing and partly because some of the tests have important predictive value for IVF outcome.

asked to be referred to the nearest IVF clinic, 40 miles away. When they went there, it seemed as if a lot of the tests were repeated again. Within a few weeks, Janet had an egg collection operation, and then the embryo transfer. When her period didn't come and her pregnancy test was positive, they couldn't believe it. They had a scan to confirm a healthy pregnancy!

With IVF for couples with unexplained infertility, the expected success rate is about 30 per cent per cycle, compared with the one to two per cent rate per cycle that is otherwise seen after three years of trying for natural conception. With three cycles of IVF or GIFT, an overall success rate of over 50 per cent should be expected if the woman is less than 40 years old.

Egg or sperm donation

Couples who are planning a family want a child using their own eggs and sperm. Sometimes, however, couples with infertility have to compromise, realising that otherwise they may not be able to fulfil their desire for a family. When couples need to consider using either eggs or sperm from someone else, it can cause an even greater sense of loss and feelings of inadequacy or failure.

If a man is donating sperm, the procedure is called donor insemination, or DI. If a woman is donating eggs, the procedure is called egg or oocyte donation. These are not treatments in the true sense of the word, but rather a means of bypassing a severe fertility problem.

WHAT ARE THE IMPLICATIONS OF TREATMENT?

For the donors
Egg or sperm donors have to go through rigorous medical screening, a detailed review of their family history, and physical and psychological testing to ensure their suitability. Both egg and sperm donation are undertaken anonymously, although, occasionally, a female friend or relative may act as an egg donor for an infertile couple.

For men who are potential sperm donors, semen and blood specimens are collected and examined for the presence of several infectious diseases, including HIV and hepatitis B and C. Once the suitability of the donor has been decided, the collection and storage of sperm may proceed. Semen samples are produced by masturbation and then freeze-stored in a liquid nitrogen 'sperm bank'. As there can be a three-month interval between acquiring an infection with HIV and the development of antibodies (which can be detected by a blood test), testing at the time of donation is not an absolute guarantee of a

REASONS FOR USING EGG OR SPERM DONATION

DONATED EGGS	DONATED SPERM
Absolute indications **for the woman – no other options** • Premature menopause (before age 40) • Surgical removal of ovaries • Absent ovaries from birth	**Absolute indications** **for the man – no other options** • Complete failure of sperm production • Vasectomy/failed vasectomy reversal
Relative indications **for the woman** • Known high risk of chromosomal or genetic abnormality • No response or very poor response to drugs at induction of ovulation or IVF • Failure of fertilisation at IVF	**Relative indications** **for the man** • Poor sperm quality (if surgical sperm collection is not possible or acceptable) • Failure of fertilisation at IVF • Known high risk of chromosomal or genetic abnormality

donor being HIV negative. For this reason, a donor is re-tested for HIV after six months, and his semen can be used for treatment only after this second HIV test is negative. The freeze–stored sperm from each individual donor can be used to father no more than ten children. The donor's physical characteristics and blood group are matched with those of the man in the couple who are being treated.

For women who are potential egg donors, similar blood tests are undertaken, particularly to exclude HIV. Once the donor is considered suitable, the preparation for egg donation can proceed. For the donor, this involves taking the usual drugs required before IVF and an egg collection operation. These procedures have small risks, and most fertility centres are reluctant to take on women whose own families are not complete. Egg donors must also be under 35 years of age, as eggs from older women carry an increased risk of abnormal chromosomal division leading to Down's syndrome. After her eggs have been collected, the donor's involvement is over and she does not require any additional drugs.

Eggs from a donor are used fresh because, unlike sperm, they do not survive freeze–storage very well. However, after they have been fertilised (usually with sperm from the husband of the recipient couple), they can be frozen and stored more successfully, to allow the necessary quarantine period for the egg donor to have repeat HIV testing. In practice, most clinics will transfer fresh embryos to the recipient woman's uterus, as these generally have a better chance of implanting than frozen embryos. The recipient woman then has to accept that this may involve a very small chance of her acquiring HIV infection. To date, there is no record of this happening in such a way.

For the infertile couple

For DI treatment, a sample of sperm is inseminated (introduced) at midcycle into the woman's cervical mucus. The timing of the procedure is obviously important and may be based on dates if her cycles are regular, or on urine hormone tests to predict ovulation if not. If donated eggs are used, the lining of the woman's uterus is prepared artificially using oestrogen and progesterone, for the transfer of embryos.

After the transfer, the drugs need to be maintained well into the pregnancy, until the placenta can function on its own (because in most cases, the primary reason for egg donation is ovarian failure, and in these women there is no

ovarian production of hormones to support the early weeks of pregnancy).

With sperm donation, the likelihood of success varies from clinic to clinic and, within individual clinics, with time. With frozen sperm, the success rate is around seven to ten per cent per cycle of treatment. In general, most clinics will suggest up to six cycles of treatment before further investigations of infertility, or other treatment options, are considered. Egg donation relies on the application of IVF techniques. In general, the supply of egg donors is not sufficient to meet the needs of the number of potential recipients. The chance of pregnancy is about 20 to 25 per cent per cycle.

The issues for any couple who wish to undergo donor treatment are complex. The use of an egg or sperm from someone else will mean the child is not genetically their own, and this can be distressing. As well as a full consultation with their specialist, couples who are considering egg or sperm donation are offered independent counselling which is also a legal requirement. If a couple feel that sperm or egg donation is too intrusive, they may consider other treatment options, such as adoption, and should be given adequate support. The issues of whom to tell and what to tell others are important, but there are no hard and fast rules. Long-term research has found that a relaxed and open approach is probably best – you may consider telling some of the following: your parents, other family members, close friends and your GP.

With regard to the legal situation, any child born within a marriage is considered a child of the marriage and the male partner is the legal father. In unmarried couples, the same is true if the male partner gives written agreement to the treatment. As this is a difficult issue, some clinics prefer to treat only married couples.

For any child born as a result of treatment

Children born as a result of DI or egg donation are accorded the full rights of any child of the family in law – including inheritance. The only exclusion to this is the inheritance of hereditary titles. For all children, their natural inquisitiveness will lead to questions:

- Who am I?
- Where did I come from?

A gradual and sensitive approach in answering these questions is necessary, particularly if they are the result of using donor eggs or sperm. You wouldn't tell a child about the rigours of labour and childbirth when they first ask these questions. Similarly, the amount of information regarding their genetic origins should fit the ability of the child's understanding. Questions shouldn't be avoided – but answers needn't be completely explicit.

Most researchers in the area would, however, suggest the child should be told – emphasising initially the specialness of the way in which they were conceived, how much their parents wanted them and what they were prepared to do to have them. How much is disclosed depends on individuals. In later life, the child may wish to know more about the donor. When they reach the age of 18, they are able to obtain non-identifying information about their genetic origins from a confidential register maintained by the Human Fertility and Embryology Authority (HFEA). This contains information such as hair colour, eye colour, likes, dislikes, family background, etc. Very occasionally, two people may wish to marry who are both the result of gamete donation – they can find out through the HFEA whether they share the same genetic mother or father, although not the identity of the individual.

KEY POINTS

✓ There are potential ethical, moral and personal difficulties that a couple need to consider before the use of donor eggs and sperm

✓ Clinics take great care to ensure close and safe matching of the donated gamete to the recipient couple

✓ Children born after the use of donated eggs or sperm are legally the children of the recipient couple

✓ Donor sperm are used only after being frozen and stored in quarantine for at least six months

✓ Donor eggs are usually freshly fertilised and the resulting embryos will be transferred without prior freeze–storage

Adoption and surrogacy

Only a small number of infertile couples need to consider adoption and surrogacy. These two options are not an easy means of achieving parenthood – both involve considerable emotional and psychological stress, as well as administrative hurdles, for the infertile couple.

ADOPTION

Adoption is the complete legal transfer of care of a child from the birth mother (or birth parents) to the adoptive parents. Most couples who consider adoption are those whose fertility treatments have failed, or who are unable to proceed with possible treatments (often for financial or religious reasons). Most of these couples would like to adopt a baby, but this is rarely possible. The introduction and widespread use of the contraceptive pill, ease of access to legal abortion and the

greater acceptance of single motherhood have all contributed to a reduction in the number of babies put forward for adoption. Although 7,342 children were adopted in the UK in 1997, only about one in ten of these were babies or children under one year of age. Adopting a young child with mental or physical disabilities may be easier, or an older child with special emotional needs. However, these children often need constant attention and can present problems for a childless couple who have no prior parenting experience.

The agencies responsible for adoption always consider the benefit for the child as their first priority, not the needs of the potential adoptive parents. A couple will be expected to have come to terms with their infertility before being considered as adoptive parents. This is to minimise the risk that the adopted child will be seen as a substitute, rather than an individual in their own right, and is one of the reasons why the process of adoption can take many months, sometimes up to two or three years.

Finding an adoption agency

There are about 200 adoption agencies in the UK. Most adoptions are arranged through local authority social services departments or through voluntary agencies such as the Catholic Children's Society, the National Children's Home or Barnardos. Information is also available from the British Agencies for Adoption and Fostering (BAAF).

Criteria for adoptive patents

There is wide regional variation in the criteria used to select potential adoptive parents. Most agencies still apply an upper age limit, usually between 34 and 40 years for both parents. Those who do not impose an upper age limit will take account of the general health of the potential adoptive parents instead. These criteria are basically for reassurance that the prospective couple will be able to provide effective parenting for a child until adulthood.

Most agencies expect a couple to be married if they want to adopt a baby. This may not be necessary for the adoption of an older child. Potential parents will be expected to have no criminal record and to be against any form of corporal punishment. Most agencies will expect both parents to have normal reading and writing abilities; this is not only so that they can deal with the large volume of literature and paperwork involved in adoption, but also so that they can support a child who may have been deprived or have learning difficulties.

The adoption process

You should write to an adoption agency with details about yourselves: your ages, how long you have been married, your race and religion, and any special skills or experience you may have. Most local authority adoption services will hold information meetings for potential parents. If the agency has vacancies on its waiting list, you will be asked to complete some formal application forms and will be allocated an adoption worker who will complete an assessment on you.

The assessment will include a police check for any past criminal record, a Social Services check for any entry on their 'at risk' register, obtaining confidential references from friends or colleagues, a medical report from your GP and any fertility clinic you have attended, and a number of home visits. The home visits give you the opportunity to discuss all aspects of adoption and enable the adoption worker to prepare a report that will be considered by an Adoption Panel. The report will include details of your family, your current relationship, and any previous relationships and lifestyle and activities, as well as exploring your feelings about your infertility, your attitudes to discipline and your expectations for your own future and that of any adopted child.

In addition to the assessment, the adoption agency will want to be certain that you are adequately prepared to take on the parenting of a child. You will usually have to attend an information and training course with other prospective couples, at evening or weekend sessions. Adoption is now a much more open process than in the past and the course will include issues such as what information to discuss with the child, and keeping records or mementoes of the birth family to maintain the child's identity if needed at a later age. Sometimes, the birth parents may ask to maintain links with their child, even after the legal transfer of care is complete. Adopted children are allowed to see their birth certificate when they reach the age of 18. Some may try to trace their genetic parents at this stage. The training course is intended to prepare prospective parents for these potentially difficult situations.

If a couple is selected by the Adoption Panel, they will go on to a waiting list for a child. There will often be some delay before a suitable child is found. The child will need to have lived with the potential adoptive parents for at least three months before they can apply to the court for an adoption order. The formal court hearing is usually brief, and the adoptive parents will be told the court's decision straight away. Once the adoption order is granted, it cannot be reversed. The child becomes a member of your family, usually takes your surname, and will inherit from you as though you were his or her birth parents.

Adopting a child from abroad

Some couples consider adopting a child from abroad. This may be because they have passed the upper age limit for local agencies in the UK, because they only feel able to accept a baby or child under the age of one year and are encountering difficulties with this in this country, or because they are moved by media attention on children who are the victims of crises or emergencies abroad. Adoption from overseas may not necessarily be in the interests of the child, can be complicated and expensive and, despite the time, cost and emotional trauma involved, may still be unsuccessful. The procedures and requirements vary from country to country.

The cost of adoption

For adoptions within the UK, the costs involved are small. Local authority adoption agencies do not charge a fee, although voluntary agencies may request a donation, as they are usually charities. Potential adoptive parents are usually required to pay a small fee for medical and police certificates. There will also be legal fees at the time of the court hearing for an adoption order, but these are also small. After an adoption order has been granted, you will be entitled to claim child benefit and any additional benefits that may be available if your child has any qualifying special needs.

If you are thinking of adopting a child from abroad, the costs can be much higher. A home study and assessment will be needed, as for a UK adoption, but you will be charged for this. The fee may be as high as £2,000 to £3,000. In addition to travelling and accommodation costs for the country from which you hope to adopt, you are likely to face high charges for local legal advice, documentation and certificates, emigration papers and possibly a donation if the child is in the care of a charitable organisation. You may need the services of an interpreter, and may also have to pay fees for translating various documents, forms and reports. The total costs of adopting from abroad can vary from £5,000 to £25,000.

SURROGACY

Surrogacy is where a host mother (the surrogate) carries a pregnancy for another couple (the commissioning or recipient couple) and gives up the baby to them after the birth. There are two main types of surrogacy. IVF surrogacy is where the pregnancy is carried by the host mother after IVF or GIFT using sperm and eggs from the commissioning couple. The pregnancy has no genetic link to the host mother and this is sometimes referred to as 'womb leasing' or 'straight surrogacy'. Variations of IVF surrogacy are where donated sperm, donated eggs or both are used.

'Natural' surrogacy is where the host mother donates her own eggs as well as carrying the pregnancy. In this situation, the surrogate is the genetic mother of the child. The pregnancy may be achieved by artificial insemination using sperm from the male partner of the commissioning couple, by intercourse with the male partner of the commissioning couple (rarely) or by artificial insemination using donor sperm.

The main indications for surrogacy are where the female

partner of the commissioning couple has been born without a uterus, where she has had to have a hysterectomy or where she has a medical condition that would be life threatening if she were to carry a pregnancy herself. Very rarely, surrogacy may be considered for couples who have had repeated miscarriages or who have had many failures to achieve a pregnancy from embryo transfer after IVF.

IVF surrogacy is only possible through clinics that are licensed to provide IVF by the Human Fertility and Embryology Authority (HFEA). A recent national survey showed that only 29 of the 115 licensed clinics in the UK provided this type of surrogacy and that only about 60 cycles of IVF surrogacy were being undertaken each year. Eggs from the female partner of the commissioning couple can be used only for IVF surrogacy if she is under the age of 35 years – the same condition that applies to egg donation.

'Natural' surrogacy is not regulated in the UK unless it involves the use of donor sperm, rather than sperm from the male partner of the commissioning couple. It is most frequently arranged by private agreement, without the involvement of a fertility clinic.

Although surrogacy is legally allowed in the UK, it is illegal for host mothers to be paid for their services by the commissioning couple. However, the commissioning couple are allowed to refund any expenses incurred by the host mother. Fertility clinics are not permitted to recruit or advertise for potential host mothers directly, and commissioning couples must find their own surrogate host independently. This may be a relative, a close friend or a volunteer who has met the commissioning couple through an introduction agency such as COTS (Childlessness Overcome Through Surrogacy).

Surrogacy raises major ethical issues and potential concerns, not least of which is the media interest and wide publicity if a host mother feels unable to give up the child. Although this occurs only rarely, it emphasises the importance of careful and extensive counselling of the commissioning couple and the host mother and her family before beginning treatment. It is also important for the commissioning couple and the host mother to have taken legal advice in advance, and to consider the need for insurance cover for any potential complications.

After the baby has been born, the commissioning couple usually take over his or her care almost immediately. It will frequently have been agreed in advance that they are present at the birth. The commissioning parents need to apply to the courts for 'Parental Orders' within six months of the birth to become the legal parents of the child. This requires the full agreement of the host mother.

KEY POINTS

✓ There are very few babies or children under one year of age available for adoption in the UK

✓ Most adoptions are arranged through local authority social service departments

✓ The process of adoption may take two to three years if a couple are eligible

✓ Adoption from abroad is complex and expensive

✓ Surrogacy treatment is only provided by about 30 clinics in the UK

✓ Payments to surrogate mothers are illegal, although expenses are allowed

Will we get a baby?

A ll couples with fertility problems want to know their chance of success with infertility treatments. This can be difficult to answer, because it depends on what is meant by 'success'. Does this mean achieving a pregnancy or having a live born baby, and should it take account of the possibility that some forms of treatment may need to be abandoned if they are not going well?

The chance of success also depends on the time-span involved and on how many cycles of treatment are undertaken. A 30 per cent chance of pregnancy within two or three months might be very acceptable, whereas a 30 per cent

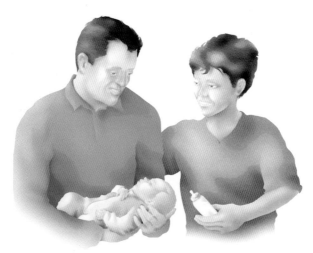

chance within two or three years would not be. There may be a number of different treatments for a couple to consider and the chance of success for each should be compared with their chance of conceiving naturally, as most couples have low fertility rather than sterility.

The experience and skill of the doctors, nurses and scientists involved in providing a fertility treatment will influence the chance of success. There can also be wide variations between different clinics. Is your chance of success based on the results in the clinic you are attending, on published results from other clinics or on nationally collected results?

Most importantly, a couple's chance of success will depend on their unique situation. Factors to consider include: their ages (particularly the woman's age); the cause of their low fertility; how carefully and thoroughly they have been investigated; whether there is more than one cause for their low fertility; the length of time that they have been trying for a pregnancy; whether they have successfully conceived in the past; their general health; and lifestyle factors such as smoking and stress. Any couple considering fertility treatment needs to know that the information that they are given about their chance of success is realistic and takes account of all these factors.

KEY POINTS

✓ Many factors need to be taken into account in estimating the chance of success with fertility treatments

✓ The woman's age is the most important factor influencing a couple's chance of conception

✓ Most fertility treatments now offer a chance of success equivalent to that of a normal fertile couple

Preparing for pregnancy

A number of health factors can reduce your chance of conceiving, increase the risk of miscarriage or increase the risk of damage to your developing baby. These risks can often be avoided or minimised by simple precautions before and during pregnancy.

RUBELLA (GERMAN MEASLES)

If you have a rubella infection in the first few weeks of pregnancy, it can affect your baby's development. You will probably have been immunised against rubella in your

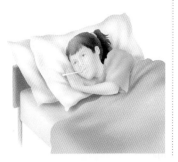

early teens. However, unlike a natural rubella infection, immunisation does not necessarily give lifelong immunity. It is therefore important that you have a blood test to check your immunity. If necessary, you will need another immunisation. As the vaccine is a weakened form of the rubella virus, you should avoid trying for a pregnancy for four weeks afterwards. You should then have a repeat blood test to check that the immunisation has been effective.

FOLIC ACID SUPPLEMENTS

If your diet is low in folic acid, you are at increased risk of conceiving a child with spina bifida or similar defects. The Department of Health now advises that all women who are planning a pregnancy should take a 400-microgram (0.4-milli-gram) folic acid supplement daily to reduce this risk. You should begin taking this about four weeks before you start to try for a baby, to build up your folic acid stores, and continue for the first 12 weeks of pregnancy. Folic acid is available over the counter at any pharmacy and in most supermarkets. You should also eat more folic acid-rich foods, such as green leafy vegetables and fortified bread or breakfast cereals. If you are taking

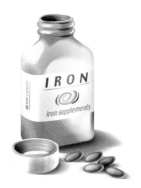

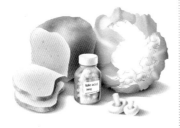

medicines for epilepsy, or you have had a previous pregnancy affected by spina bifida, consult your GP, as you may need to take a higher dose of folic acid (five milligrams daily).

DIET AND FOOD HYGIENE

A healthy well-balanced diet is important while you are trying to conceive and during pregnancy. If you are vegetarian, you may have reduced reserves of iron, which is mainly found in red meat. You may

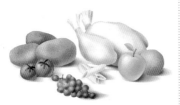

need to have a blood test to check this before trying for a pregnancy, in case you need to take iron supplements.

Caffeine-containing drinks (coffee, tea and Coca-Cola, for example) taken in above-average amounts can reduce the fertility of men and women. Limit your consumption of these drinks to no

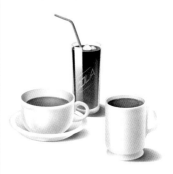

more than six cups daily or change to decaffeinated equivalents.

You will need to avoid certain foods during fertility treatment and pregnancy. These include soft, ripened cheeses, especially those made with unpasteurised or raw milk, as these may carry a small risk of infections (such as *Listeria*) that can lead to miscarriage. Liver and liver products (such as pâtés) should also be avoided. These contain very high levels of vitamin A, which can lead to abnormalities in a developing baby. For the same reason, don't take food supplements containing vitamin A.

Basic food hygiene is important to minimise any risk of food poisoning. Cook meat and poultry thoroughly and avoid seafood and shellfish. When using a microwave oven for reheating food, make sure the food is piping hot all the way through. Use a separate knife and board for meat and poultry, and clean any work surfaces and wash your hands thoroughly before and after food preparation. Keep raw and cooked foods separate, preferably wrapped or in containers. Store raw meat on the lowest shelf of your refrigerator to avoid juices dripping onto other cooked food.

Some women who are overweight, particularly those with polycystic ovarian syndrome, will be

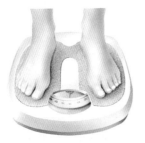

able to improve their chance of pregnancy and reduce their risk of miscarriage by losing weight. Women who are underweight can also increase their chance of conceiving and minimise their risk of pregnancy complications by gaining weight.

TOXOPLASMOSIS AND CHLAMYDIA

Toxoplasmosis is a mild infection in most people. However, if it is passed from a mother to her developing baby during pregnancy, it can cause severe damage, particularly to the baby's eyes and brain. The parasites called *Toxoplasma* that cause the infection can be carried by cats, dogs and

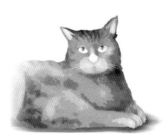

sheep. If you have a cat, don't handle or change soiled litter. If this is unavoidable, wear rubber gloves and wash your hands afterwards. You should also wear gloves during gardening, and wash your hands afterwards, as soil can be contaminated with *Toxoplasma*. Even if your cat or dog is clean and healthy, you should wash your hands after handling them or their food bowls.

Chlamydia causes a sexually transmitted disease. Although it doesn't always cause symptoms, it can block or damage the fallopian tubes, leading to infertility problems. It may also be responsible for an ectopic pregnancy (when a fertilised egg implants in the fallopian tubes, rather than in the uterus), which can be life threatening. *Chlamydia* can affect the health of a baby, causing conjunctivitis of the eyes and possibly pneumonia. If you think you are at risk of chlamydia infection, ask your GP for advice. It can be treated with antibiotics.

SMOKING AND ALCOHOL

A couple's chance of conceiving naturally, or with fertility treatment, is greater if they are both non-smokers, avoid passive smoking and limit their alcohol intake to no more than 6 units weekly or better still, to none at all.

DRUGS AND MEDICAL CONDITIONS

It is best to avoid any drugs during pregnancy, particularly during the first few weeks when most of the important organs in your baby will be developing. If you are taking any medicines, it is important to check with your GP or local fertility clinic that these are not potentially harmful or likely to reduce your fertility.

If you have a chronic medical condition, you may need to have your treatment reviewed or adjusted, before trying for a pregnancy. This is particularly important if you have diabetes, epilepsy, thyroid disease, heart disease or a blood-clotting disorder. In addition, some drug treatments for arthritic problems can reduce your fertility and may need to be altered. You should seek advice from your GP.

Recreational drugs should be avoided while you are trying to conceive and during pregnancy. In

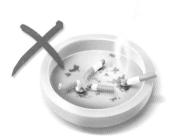
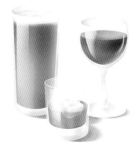

Both tobacco and alcohol consumption reduce the chances of conceiving.

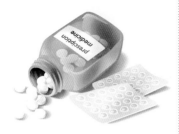

particular, cannabis can interfere with ovulation and cocaine crosses the placenta and may lead to addiction for the unborn baby.

FOREIGN TRAVEL

If you plan to travel abroad during pregnancy or fertility treatment, you'll need to take precautions, particularly with your diet and food hygiene. Some immunisations, such as those for yellow fever, cholera, typhoid and poliomyelitis, use modified live material and should be used only if the risk of infection is high at your destination. In addition, some anti-malarial drugs (such as primaquine and maloprim) are best avoided; with others (such as pyrimethamine), you may need to take a higher dose of folic acid. However, the benefits of preventing malaria greatly outweigh the risk from the disease, and there are alternative safe drugs. Ask your GP or clinic nurse for advice.

KEY POINTS

✓ Plan for your pregnancy in advance by adjusting your diet, optimising your weight and adopting a healthy lifestyle

✓ Check your rubella immunity and start taking folic acid supplements

✓ Stop smoking and restrict your alcohol intake

✓ Pay extra attention to food hygiene

✓ Check with your GP if you have any medical condition or are taking any medicines regularly

Coping with infertility

Most couples with fertility problems go through a stressful experience. Some will ultimately be successful and will move on from this phase of their life. There will, however, be some couples who will never manage to have a child. In some way, they have to learn to cope with the situation and to carry on with their lives.

In many respects, these couples are experiencing a loss or absence, focusing on the children they are unable to have. Some cope well with all of this, others not so well. The support and understanding of family and close friends can be invaluable but, sadly, this is not always available. Couples who have not experienced the emotional pain of childlessness themselves may find it difficult to understand the depth and duration of the sadness it causes.

Genuine depression will be a problem for some couples and may require medical treatment. For others, infertility can lead to difficulties in their relationship and professional counselling may be necessary.

Coming to terms with not having children can take many years. Sometimes, this adjustment will be easier if a couple feels that they have done everything possible to achieve a pregnancy, even if this means a final attempt at a treatment that has a very low chance of success. Infertility clinic nurses and doctors try to help people cope with their infertility. The difficult decision to stop treatment can sometimes liberate a couple to get on with their lives.

It is important for couples to recognise that their inability to conceive should not affect how they view themselves as men or women and is not a reflection of their sexual activity. Men with sperm problems often experience anxiety and emotional difficulties because of confusion between fertility and virility. A man with a very low or absent sperm count will still be producing normal levels of testosterone and other male hormones. His masculinity and sexual potency will be the same as for any other man.

KEY POINTS

✓ Fertility problems are a stressful experience

✓ Some couples will never manage to have a child

✓ Sometimes coming to terms with not having children will be made easier if a couple feel that they have done everything possible to achieve a pregnancy

✓ The difficult decision to stop treatment can liberate a couple to carry on with the rest of their lives

Useful addresses

UK INTERNET WEBSITES

Centre for Reproductive Medicine
University of Bristol
www.repromed.org.uk/crm

The Bridge Centre
www.thebridgecentre.co.uk

The Human Fertilisation and Embryology Authority
www.hfea.gov.uk

The Royal College of Obstetricians and Gynaecologists
www.rcog.org.uk

ASSOCIATIONS

British Agencies for Adoption and Fostering (BAAF)
Head Office
Skyline House
200 Union Street
London SE1 0LX
Tel: 020 7593 2000
Fax: 020 7593 2001
Email: mail@baaf.org.uk
Website: www.baaf.org.uk

This association coordinates adoption agencies, provides information and a list of children awaiting adoption or fostering.

British Infertility Counselling Association (BICA)
69 Division Street
Sheffield S1 4GE
Tel: 01342 843880

This association provides a list of counsellors who deal with fertility problems.

CHILD (The National Infertility Support Network)
Charter House, 3 St Leonard's Road
Bexhill-on-Sea
East Sussex TN40 1JA
Tel: 01424 732361
Fax: 01424 731858
Website: www.child.org.uk

This network provides information, advice and a list of local support groups.

Childlessness Overcome Through Surrogacy (COTS)
Loandhu Cottage
Gruidas
Lairg, Sutherland
Scotland IV27 4EF
Tel: 01549 402401
Fax: 01549 402777

This association runs a surrogacy helpline.

Daisy Network
PO Box 392
High Wycombe
Bucks HP15 7SH
Email: info@daisynetwork.org.uk
Website: www.daisychain.org

The Daisy Network (previously known as the Daisy Chain) is a support group for women suffering premature menopause. Exchanges information on IVF, HRT and on ways to have a family through egg donation, surrogacy or adoption. Provides informal telephone counselling by members and a quarterly newsletter.

DI Network
PO Box 265
Sheffield S3 7YX
Tel/fax: 0181 245 4369
Website: www.issue.co.uk/dinet

This national network provides social and emotional support for families with children conceived with donated gametes.

Home Office
Immigration and Nationality Department
Lunar House
Wellesley Road
Croydon
Surrey CR9 2BY
Tel: 08706 067766

The Home Office produces a document (Circular RON 117) that explains the entry requirements for children who are being brought into the UK for adoption.

Human Fertilisation and Embryology Authority (HFEA)
Paxton House
30 Artillery Lane
London E1 7LS
Tel: 020 7377 5077
Fax: 020 7377 1871
Website: www.hfea.gov.uk

This statutory government body regulates clinics providing IVF, donor insemination and embryo research. It produces an annual Patient's Guide, with extensive information about all licensed IVF centres in the UK (including their success rates).

Independent Fertility Concerns Resource Centre
44 Eversden Road
Harlton
Cambridge CB3 7ET
Tel: 01223 262226
Fax: 01223 264332
Website: www.ifc.co.uk/info.htm/

Provides information for patients and the public in the form of CD-Roms and children's books to help parents tell their children about their conception.

ISSUE (The National Fertility Association)
114 Lichfield Street
Walsall WS1 1SZ
Tel: 01922 722888
Fax: 01922 640070
Email: webmaster@issue.co.uk
Website: www.issue.co.uk

This association provides support for people with fertility problems.

Miscarriage Association

c/o Clayton Hospital
Northgate
Wakefield
West Yorkshire WF1 3JS
Tel: 01924 200799
Fax: 01924 298834
Scottish helpline (answerphone): 0131 334 8883
Website: www.btinternet.com/~miscarriage.association

Provides support and information on all aspects of pregnancy loss.

Multiple Births Foundation

Queen Charlotte's & Chelsea Hospital
Goldhawk Road
London W6 9XG
Tel: 0181 383 3519
Fax: 0181 383 3041
Email: mbf@rpms.ac.uk
Website: www.multiplebirths.org.uk

The foundation provides support for families with multiple births.

National Endometriosis Society

50 Westminster Palace Gardens
Artillery Row
London SW1P 1RL
Helpline: 020 7222 2776 (7–10pm)
Tel: 020 7222 2781
Fax: 020 7222 2786
Email: endo webmaster@dial.pipex.com
Website: www.endo.org.uk

This society provides support, information and advice for women with endometriosis.

National Infertility Awareness Campaign (NIAC)

PO Box 2106
London W1A 3DZ
Helpline: 0800 716345
Tel: 020 7439 3067

Overseas Adoption Helpline

PO Box 13899
London N6 4WB
Helpline: 0990 168742
Fax: 0181 348 1522

Provides information on overseas adoption.

TAMBA (Twins & Multiple Births Association)

Harnott House
309 Chester Road
Little Sutton
South Wirral L66 1TH
Helpline: 01732 868000 (7–11pm weekdays, 10am–11pm weekends)
Tel: 0151 348 0020 or 0870 121 4000
Fax: 0870 121 4001 or 0151 348 0765
Email: tamba@information4u.com
Website: www.surreyweb.org.uk/tamba/

This is a national confidential support and information service for all parents of multiple births.

Glossary

Adhesion: a band of scar tissue in the abdomen, which usually results from an infection or other tissue damage.

Amenorrhoea: the complete absence or cessation of menstrual periods.

Anovulation: the failure to ovulate.

Azoospermia: the complete absence of sperm in seminal fluid.

Cervical mucus: the thick clear fluid produced from the cervix, which becomes thinner just before ovulation.

Cervix: the fibrous circular structure at the lower end of the uterus, often called the 'neck of the womb'.

Chlamydia: a bacterium that is generally transmitted as a result of sexual intercourse, which can infect, damage and block the fallopian tubes.

Chromosomes: the 46 tiny strands of genes that are contained in every cell in the body and control their function. One half of these are inherited from each parent. Down's syndrome is an example of a chromosomal abnormality.

Clomiphene citrate: a drug (given in tablet form) to induce ovulation.

Conception: the process of becoming pregnant.

Donor insemination (DI): artificial insemination using donor sperm.

Ectopic pregnancy: a pregnancy where the embryo has implanted outside the woman's uterus, usually in one of her fallopian tubes.

Egg (oocyte): a cell produced by the ovary that contains half the normal amount of genetic material (and which fuses with the male sperm at fertilisation to produce an embryo).

Embryo: the developing fertilised egg from the time of fertilisation until organ development is complete (at about ten weeks of pregnancy).

Endometriosis: a condition in which tissue resembling the lining of the uterus is present in the pelvis.

Endometrium/endometrial lining: soft tissue produced in the uterus every month into which the developing embryo implants.

Epididymis (pl. epididymes): the tightly coiled tube on the surface of the testis where sperm mature before they are released by ejaculation.

Fallopian tube: a round tube with finger-like projections at its outer end that pick up the egg at ovulation and through which the sperm pass to reach and fertilise the egg. The resulting embryo passes down the fallopian tube to reach the cavity of the uterus.

Fertilisation: the union of a sperm and an egg that results in an embryo.

Fetus: the fully formed developing organism from the tenth week of pregnancy onwards to the time of birth.

Fibroid: a benign muscle growth in the wall of the uterus.

Fimbria(e): the finger-like structure at the outer ends of the fallopian tubes, nearest to the ovaries, which attaches to the ovaries and traps the egg as it is released, directing it into the fallopian tubes.

Follicle: a fluid-filled area in the ovaries that grows in each menstrual cycle and produces a mature egg capable of fertilisation.

FSH (follicle-stimulating hormone): a hormone produced by the pituitary gland that acts on the ovaries to stimulate follicle growth.

Gamete: a sperm or an egg.

GIFT (gamete intrafallopian transfer): a procedure involving egg collection and the immediate surgical placement of up to three eggs and prepared sperm directly into a fallopian tube.

GnRH (gonadotrophin-releasing hormone): a hormone produced by the hypothalamus that stimulates the pituitary gland to produce FSH and LH.

Gonadotrophin: a hormone, such as FSH or LH, that stimulates the ovaries or testes.

hCG (human chorionic gonadotrophin): a hormone that is similar to LH and is used to stimulate ovulation during fertility drug treatments.

hMG (human menopausal gonadotrophin): a hormone extracted from the urine of post-menopausal women that contains FSH and LH and is given by injections to induce ovulation.

Hormone: a chemical produced in one part of the body that acts in another part. For example, FSH produced in the pituitary gland stimulates the ovaries to produce an egg.

HSG (hysterosalpingography): a procedure in which dye is passed through the uterus into the fallopian tubes, which can then be seen on X-ray.

Hydrosalpinx (pl. hydrosalpinges): a collection of fluid secretions inside a blocked fallopian tube.

Hypothalamus: the central part of the brain that controls many body hormones and secretes GnRH.

Hysteroscopy: direct visual inspection of the cavity of the uterus using a small telescopic instrument, under general or local anaesthesia.

ICSI (intracytoplasmic sperm injection): the technique in which an individual sperm is injected into the nucleus of an individual egg, usually as a treatment for male infertility.

Insemination: the addition of sperm either into the woman's uterus through the cervix or in the laboratory to eggs for IVF.

IUI (intrauterine insemination): a process in which prepared sperm are placed at the top of the uterine cavity, usually at the time of (artificially induced) ovulation.

IVF (in vitro fertilisation): a procedure involving egg collection, preparation of sperm and then a mixture of the two; the eggs are inspected some hours later to check for signs of fertilisation and then allowed to develop further outside the body until they can be transferred back into the uterus two or three days later.

Laparoscopy: an operation requiring an anaesthetic and involving the passage of a small telescope-like instrument into the abdomen, allowing direct visual inspection of the internal genital organs, an assessment of the fallopian tubes and of disease processes such as endometriosis.

LH (luteinising hormone): a hormone produced by the pituitary gland that acts on the ovary to stimulate egg release (ovulation).

Menopause: the end of menstruation, usually around the age of 50, when the supply of a woman's own eggs in her ovaries is exhausted. The production of oestrogen from the ovaries also falls at this time giving the symptoms of the menopause.

Miscarriage: loss of pregnancy before the fetus is capable of surviving outside the uterus (before 24 weeks of pregnancy).

Oestrogen: the main female hormone produced by the ovaries from the cells in the wall of developing follicles.

Oocyte: an egg produced by the ovary and which contains half the normal amount of genetic material (and which fuses with the male sperm at fertilisation to produce an embryo).

Ovary: one of two organs in the woman's pelvis that produce an egg every month and the hormones oestrogen and progesterone.

Ovulation: the process in which an egg is released from an ovary in the middle of a woman's monthly cycle after stimulation (usually by the body's own hormones), and an essential step to getting pregnant.

PCO (polycystic ovaries): a condition in which the ovaries contain many small non-cancerous cysts (which are actually immature egg follicles rather than true cysts). Additional symptoms include weight gain, irregular periods, infertility, acne, increased body hair growth and an increased risk of miscarriage. When those additional symptoms are present, it is usually referred to as polycystic ovarian syndrome (PCOS).

PCT (postcoital test): an infertility investigation in which the woman's cervical mucus is collected and examined microscopically a few hours after intercourse to check that sperm are present.

Pituitary: a small, pea-sized structure at the base of the brain that releases a wide range of hormones, particularly FSH and LH.

Placenta: also called the afterbirth. An important structure connected to the wall of the uterus, and by the umbilical cord to the baby. It permits nutrients and oxygen to reach the baby and waste products to leave the baby, and also has an important function in hormone production to maintain the pregnancy.

Progesterone: a hormone produced in the second half of the woman's menstrual cycle after ovulation. It is crucial to the maintenance of an early pregnancy before the placenta begins to function.

Rubella: German measles, a generally mild illness in a woman. If it develops in the first half of pregnancy, it can have serious consequences for the baby, possibly causing blindness or deafness.

Semen (seminal fluid): the carrier fluid, including sperm, released by a man at ejaculation.

Seminal vesicles: the organs in which seminal fluid is added to sperm to help carry the sperm into the vagina and cervix.

Seminiferous tubules: the tiny tubes in the testes where sperm are formed.

Sperm: the tiny cells present in the fluid that a man ejaculates at orgasm. Sperm can unite with an egg to form an embryo. Produced by the male in the seminiferous tubules of the testis, they contain half of the normal genetic content of the man.

Spermatogenesis: the process in which sperm are produced in the testis.

SSR (surgical sperm recovery): a procedure in which sperm are collected directly from the man's testes or epididymes for ICSI when he produces no sperm in his ejaculate.

Testis/testicle (pl. testes): one of the two organs in the male, found in the scrotum, which are responsible for the production of sperm and testosterone, the principal male sex hormone.

Urethra: the passageway connected to the bladder that allows urine to leave the body. It allows the release of semen from the penis through a number of small openings just below the bladder.

Uterus (the womb): the muscular organ in the centre of a woman's pelvis where a pregnancy is carried.

Vas deferens: a thin cord-like structure, which can easily be felt above the testicle in the scrotum, along which sperm are released from the testicle and epididymis.

Zona pellucida: the tough, outer covering of the egg.

Zygote: the fertilised egg.

Index